THE MONOGRAPH SERIES OF
THE PSYCHOANALYTIC STUDY OF THE CHILD

Monograph No. 2

EARLY CHILDHOOD DISTURBANCES,
THE INFANTILE NEUROSIS,
AND THE ADULTHOOD DISTURBANCES

Problems of a Developmental Psychoanalytic Psychology

THE PSYCHOANALYTIC STUDY OF THE CHILD
MONOGRAPH NO. 2

Early Childhood Disturbances,
the Infantile Neurosis, and the Adulthood
Disturbances

Problems of a Developmental Psychoanalytic Psychology

By

HUMBERTO NAGERA, M.D.

The Hampstead Child-Therapy Clinic, London

INTERNATIONAL UNIVERSITIES PRESS, INC.
NEW YORK

THE MONOGRAPH SERIES OF
THE PSYCHOANALYTIC STUDY OF THE CHILD

Managing Editors

Ruth S. Eissler, M.D.   Heinz Hartmann, M.D.

Anna Freud, LL.D., Sc.D.   Marianne Kris, M.D.

Editorial Assistant

Lottie M. Newman

All contributions for publication in the Monograph Series will be by invitation only. The Editors regret that they do not have facilities to read unsolicited manuscripts.

To Anna Freud

CONTENTS

Foreword by Anna Freud   9

Acknowledgments   11

1. The Background for a Developmental
   Psychoanalytic Psychology   13
2. The Concept of "Infantile Neurosis"   20
3. Developmental Interference   28
4. Developmental Conflicts   41
5. Neurotic Conflicts   48
6. The Infantile Neurosis   54
7. Differences and Similarities between the
   Infantile and the Adult Neurosis: With
   Some Comments on Prediction   63
8. Childhood Disturbances as the Basis of
   Adulthood Disturbances   72
9. A Developmental Scheme: Toward Normality,
   Neurosis or Other Forms of Disturbance   77

Bibliography   85

Index   89

About the Author   95

7

FOREWORD

Dr. H. Nagera's monograph bears witness to the child analyst's dissatisfaction with the present mode of diagnostic thinking. As stated by him, we are not content any longer to subsume all childhood disorders under the all-embracing title of an "infantile neurosis," as analysts tended to do in former eras of psychoanalysis. Nor do we consider it an adequate solution to search for our answer to all diagnostic questions in any one period of childhood, whether late, in the oedipal phase, as the classical view sets out, or early in the first year of life, as more recent views assert. Nor are we ready to accept the exclusive indictment of either faulty object relationships or faulty ego development, which many modern authors treat as the only potential sources of trouble.

What the author of this monograph does to remedy the position is a careful apportioning of pathogenic impact to external and internal interferences at any time of the child's life; the location of the internal influences in any part of the psychic structure or in the interaction between any of the inner agencies; and the building up, step by step, of an orderly sequence of childhood disorders, of which the infantile neurosis is not the base, but the final, complex apex.

What satisfies the student of analysis in an exposition of

this nature is the fact that on the one hand it is rooted in the notion of a hypothetical norm of childhood development, while on the other hand it establishes a hierarchy of disturbances which is valid for the period of immaturity and meaningful as a forerunner of adult psychopathology.

Anna Freud

London, September 1965

ACKNOWLEDGMENTS

This monograph forms part of a study entitled "Assessment of Pathology in Childhood," which is conducted at the Hampstead Child-Therapy Clinic and Course, London. It has been financed by the National Institute of Mental Health, Washington.

The monograph could never have been written but for the stimulating psychoanalytic climate of the Hampstead Clinic. Thus the writer is in debt to all its members, but especially to those who kindly have given permission to use examples from their case material collected in different departments.

Special thanks are due to Dr. L. Frankl and Dr. J. Bolland (Diagnostic Department), Dr. J. Stross (Well-Baby Clinic), Miss A. Bene and Mrs. M. Friedman (Educational Unit), and Mrs. M. Burgner, Miss A. Colonna, Mrs. E. Dansky, Miss R. Edgcumbe, Mr. W. Ernest Freud, Miss G. Jones, Miss R. Putzel, Miss K. Ress, and Mrs. L. Weitzner, all members of the "Clinical Concept Research Group" with whom I have been able to discuss some aspects of this monograph and from whom I have received much constructive criticism.

Finally, to Miss Nancy Procter-Gregg and Mrs. Lottie M. Newman, who have corrected the English style and made many valuable suggestions.

To all many thanks.

11

CHAPTER 1

THE BACKGROUND
FOR A DEVELOPMENTAL
PSYCHOANALYTIC PSYCHOLOGY

In 1950 Ernst Kris wrote: "There seems to be wide agreement that the psychoanalytical study of child development would fill an urgent need, might usefully function as a center of integration of various approaches and promises the only way to answer the questions with which we are all occupied, questions in which the problem of prevention is omnipresent" (p. 37). I think every analyst will agree with this statement. Further, by now a great deal of work has already been done by a large number of analysts. It seems a good time to take stock of the many contributions concerning different aspects and areas of a developmental psychoanalytic psychology. While an attempt to review and integrate all the findings is beyond the scope of this presentation, it is clear that their close examination would at least highlight the present position of psychoanalysis in these respects and indicate possible ways for future development and research.

My central aim is an attempt to scrutinize the current concept of "infantile neurosis," to focus on its central position in normal and abnormal development, and to examine its similarities to and differences from the adulthood disturbances. I shall also describe different forms of early disturbances in children which I believe should not be referred to as neurosis, although these disturbances produce symptoms which in many ways are similar to those produced by the conflicts observed in the neuroses. Furthermore, these early forms of disturbance do play a most important role in the later development toward normality, neurosis, or any other form of adult psychopathology.

Before embarking on a discussion of my central topics I shall briefly review a number of the basic assumptions underlying the psychoanalytic developmental psychology. These views form the background of the approach used in this study.

The term "development" is here used in the widest possible sense to include both physical and psychological development. Similarly the term "maturation" can cover both physical and psychological maturation. This usage is different from that of Hartmann, Kris, and Loewenstein (1946).

Because the central nervous system of the human infant is quite immature at birth, some of the basic organic structures necessary for the performance of many complex functions are not yet developed. These functions cannot properly be performed until the physical maturation required has been completed. Thus, at this early stage there exists the closest relationship between actual physical maturational development (especially of the central nervous system) and psychological development. With the progress of physical maturation, psychological development increasingly takes leave of its organic ties.[1] It now develops in its own right to great heights of sophistication and complexity. It seems that with the achievement of the basic physical maturation a given potential for psychological development has been laid down. How far the latter will reach is now largely dependent on phenomena of a psychological nature—taking in part at least the form of specific stimuli from the environment and the interaction with the objects.

Hartmann (1950a) too has pointed out that the "problem

[1] This is of course a relative statement. The integrity of the anatomical structure remains a *sine qua non* condition for the performance of its function.

of maturation has a physiological aspect. . . . We have to assume that differences in the timing or intensity of their growth enter into the picture of ego development as a partly independent variable; e.g., the timing of the appearance of grasping, of walking, of the motor aspect of speech" (p. 80). Hartmann, Kris, and Loewenstein further stated (1946, p. 18): "Differentiation and integration in the child's early phases of development are partly regulated by maturational sequence, but even where they are influenced by environmental conditions, we are compelled to assume a principle regulating their interaction (Hartmann, 1939)."

Very generally speaking, psychoanalysis assumes that psychological unfolding results from the interaction between internal and external factors. While some aspects of development are closely connected with conflict situations, other aspects belong to what Hartmann (1939) refers to as the "conflict-free ego sphere."

> After all, mental development is not simply the outcome of the struggle with instinctual drives, with love-objects, with the superego, and so on. For instance, we have reason to assume that this development is served by apparatuses which function from the beginning of life; . . . For now, we will mention only that memory, associations, and so on, are functions which cannot possibly be derived from the ego's relationships to instinctual drives or love-objects, but are rather *prerequisites* of our conception of these and of their development [p. 15]. We must recognize that though the ego certainly does grow on conflicts, these are not the only roots of ego development. Many of us expect psychoanalysis to become a general *developmental psychology:* to do so, it must encompass these other roots of ego development, by reanalyzing from its own point of view and with its own methods the results obtained in these areas by nonanalytic psychology. . . .
>
> [He further pointed out:] Not every adaptation to the environment, or every learning and maturation process, is a conflict. I refer to the development *outside of conflict* of perception, intention, object comprehension, thinking, language, recall-phenomena, productivity, to the well-known phases of

motor development, grasping, crawling, walking, and to the maturation and learning processes implicit in all these and many others [pp. 7-8].

Furthermore, Hartmann emphasized the need to study the possible interactions of the different and otherwise somewhat independent developmental processes. He said:

> Our task is to investigate how mental conflict and "peaceful" internal development mutually facilitate and hamper each other. We must, likewise, study the interplay between conflict and that aspect of development with which we are familiar mostly from its relations to the external world. Thus, to take a simple example, learning to walk upright combines constitution, maturation of the apparatus, and learning processes, with those libidinal processes, identifications, endogenous and exogenous (instinctual drive and environmental) factors which may lead to conflicts and to disturbances of function [p. 11].
> In our clinical work we observe daily how differences in intellectual development, in motor development, and so on, affect the child's coping with conflicts and how this in turn influences intellectual and motor development. Such observations establish descriptively the interaction of the conflict-sphere with other ego functions [p. 16].

Hartmann restated some of these views in the Introduction to his book, *Essays on Ego Psychology* (1964). After referring to Freud's suggestion (1937) that not only the instinctual drives but also the ego might have a hereditary core, Hartmann states:

> I think we have the right to assume that there are, in man, inborn apparatuses which I have called primary autonomy, and that these primary autonomous apparatuses of the ego and their maturation constitute one foundation for the relations to external reality. Among those factors originating in the hereditary core of the ego, there are also those which serve postponement of discharge, that is, which are of an inhibitory nature. . . . On the other hand, many, though not all, ego activities can be traced genetically to determinants in the id or to conflicts between ego and id. In the course of development, however, they

normally acquire a certain amount of autonomy from these genetic factors. The ego's achievements may under some circumstances be reversible, but it is important to know that in normal conditions many of them are not. . . . We speak of the degrees of this independence of the ego as the degrees of secondary autonomy [p. xi].

Kris (1950) said that we now have a better understanding of the extent to which conflict, danger, and defense are part and parcel of normal development; in fact, they are essential and necessary concomitants of growing up, as Anna Freud (1945) has shown. He further referred to the suggestion by Hartmann, Kris, and Loewenstein (1946) that the future development of autonomous ego functions is related not to the absence of conflict but to an optimal distance from conflict.

It is a generally accepted assumption that development can proceed normally only under certain ideal conditions of which we are on the whole quite ignorant. We are forced to conclude that whatever these ideal conditions may be, they allow for very wide variations.

Anything departing too far[2] from these norms constitutes an "interference" with the conditions under which development ought to have proceeded. We give the name of "developmental interferences" to any happenings, situations, conditions, or events of this sort. They tend to enforce, especially when they are very marked, some sort of readjustment or redirection of the developmental processes.

Freud (1914) put forward the hypothesis that "The development of the ego consists in a departure from primary narcissism and gives rise to a vigorous attempt to recover that state." Similarly, I believe that some aspects of human development are due to the frustration of the primary needs of the newborn infant. Such frustrations are inevitable even in the presence of ideal conditions and ideal mothering (see,

[2] Too far implies either quantitative or qualitative factors beyond certain points tolerable for the developing organism.

for example, Anna Freud, 1954). Disturbances of the basic
homeostatic equilibrium of the primitive organism forced
development forward with the essential aim of recovering the
basic state of inner equilibrium, the hypothetical state of
primary narcissism. Complete satisfaction would have made
development from the original state unnecessary. The types
of conflict here being referred to are not necessarily neurotic
conflicts but rather conflicts around "adaptation" to the new
conditions (extra-uterine). At later stages adaptive processes
and the conflicts pertaining to them concern, as Hartmann
(1939) pointed out, both processes connected with conflict
situations and processes relating to the conflict-free sphere.

In any case development as outlined above implies multiple processes acting independently as well as simultaneously
interacting in the more diverse ways.

Protection from excessive stimulation plays an important
role. On the other hand, specific forms of ego and drive
stimulation are essential for development to proceed along
adequate paths. This has been demonstrated by a number of
analysts, notably so by Spitz and Wolf (1946), Anna Freud
and Dann (1951), and most recently by Provence and Lipton
in their interesting book *Infants in Institutions* (1962). Experiencing and learning are two other essential factors con-
tributing to the development of the total personality and
especially of the ego aspects of it.

It is not always easy to foresee the ways in which different
developmental influences will direct development. They can
either further it or hinder it. Anna Freud (1936) has shown
that in some cases anxiety of a certain intensity stimulates
intelligence. Helene Deutsch (1944) demonstrated that phases
of intense conflict such as prepuberty may tend to favor
progressive trends. Furthermore, the same event may in some
children act as a stimulus to further development, while in
others it has a retarding, hindering effect.

These deviations can occur in all sorts of directions—on the

side of the drives, the ego, the superego, and the object relationships.[3]

Similarly, different developmental phases require different
ideal conditions, and certain events or interferences are especially significant if they take place at a certain developmental
stage. Furthermore, it largely depends on the developmental
stage of children what aspect of some not uncommon but
nevertheless disturbing events will be of significance for any
given child. For example, a tonsillectomy performed at the
peak of the phallic-oedipal phase will frequently reinforce
the child's castration anxiety and may be of special significance in this context as a punishment for the oedipal fantasies and accompanying masturbatory activities. For a
younger child who has not yet reached this phase, the most
traumatic and significant element of the same event may be
the separation involved in the hospitalization.

An event which influences development will show its effect
not only at the time of its occurrence but will frequently also
act as a disturbance at a much later time when the child is at
a different developmental stage. Thus, in one of our cases,
the sudden death of the father while the child was going
through the anal-sadistic stage brought about an important
fixation at this point in the child's development. This fixation in turn influenced the course of his later development
and played an important role in the intensity and in the form
of expression of his infantile neurosis. By the time the child
had moved into the phallic-oedipal position the absence of a
"real father" made it easier for him to give free rein to his
fantasy without any possible check in reality. Thus, the usual
conflicts of the oedipal stage were further complicated and
their resolution became more difficult and troublesome.

---

[3] Here considered as a function of the interaction of drives, ego (superego)
development of a subject (the baby, the child, the adult) with the drives and
ego (superego) interaction of the object (the mother to start with, and later on
whoever that object may be).

CHAPTER 2

THE CONCEPT OF "INFANTILE NEUROSIS"

In recent years the concept of "infantile neurosis" has slowly been displaced from its central position in psychoanalytic thinking. In some cases, as in Melanie Klein's formulations, it has disappeared altogether; if it is referred to at all, the infantile neurosis is considered to be a defensive structure. I believe that the concept should remain a central one in "psychoanalytic psychology."

Some of the reasons for this gradual displacement were discussed at a special meeting devoted to "Problems of Infantile Neurosis" (see Kris et al., 1954). On this occasion Hartmann stated his belief "that most of what Freud said about infantile neurosis long ago remains true today" (p. 32). However, he added: "It is actually not so easy to say what we call an infantile neurosis" (p. 33). He reminded us that when Freud first approached this problem, he found that what he regarded a neurosis was frequently taken to be naughtiness and bad upbringing by teachers and parents. Hartmann pointed to the swing in the opposite direction today when "every naughtiness, actually every behavior of the child that does not conform to the textbook model, every developmental step that is not according to plan, is considered as 'neurotic'" (p. 33). He considered the implications of such a swing, answering in the following way: "It means that the broad range of normal

20

variations of behavior is not recognized, and that the specific features of what analysts call a neurosis get lost." He continued with the following extremely important comment: "Apart from this, however, many of the very early neuroses are really different from what we are used to calling neurosis in the adult. Many problems in children which we call neurotic are actually limited to a single functional disturbance; and the way from conflict to symptom seems often to be shorter than in adult neurosis" (p. 33).

More than one of the discussants at the "Problems of Infantile Neurosis" symposium pointed out that very little was in fact being said about the infantile neurosis. Hartmann commented: "You will have noticed that in both Dr. Greenacre's and Miss Freud's paper, relatively little has been said about infantile neurosis proper, which is of course significant for the state of affairs today" (p. 32). Anna Freud similarly pointed out that the contributions to the symposium were "concerned mainly with one aspect of [the infantile neurosis], namely with the earliest possible pathogenic influences which date back to the child's first year of life" (p. 25).[1]

The issues discussed at the symposium can, to the best of my knowledge, be considered to be fairly representative of the problems and difficulties found in this area. The position has not changed very much since 1954. If anything I would say that the concept of infantile neurosis has become even more obscured and has gradually been displaced from the central position it should occupy.

Many factors have in different ways contributed to the lack of precision in our formulations and in our understanding of the infantile neurosis and earlier forms of disturbances, as well as to the increasing obscurity and confusion in this respect.

Psychoanalysis began with the study of neurosis in the adult. Freud made his essential observations in this specific field, and it is therefore readily understandable that his for-

[1] Freud's views of the infantile neurosis are described in detail in Chapters 5 and 6.

mulations were particularly suitable for the explanation of
this type of disturbance. However, it soon became clear that
the differences between the neuroses and the ideal norm were
mostly a quantitative matter and that the psychoanalytic
model was equally suitable for the study of normal psychological processes. Psychoanalysis was thus transformed into a
psychoanalytic psychology. With "the widening scope of psychoanalysis,"[2] many other forms of disturbances were also
studied with the new conceptual tool. Some of these disturbances—and especially certain aspects of them—differed from
the normal not merely in quantitative terms, as had been the
case in the neuroses. In some of these disturbances there were
essential differences of a genetic and developmental nature.

Not all that is observed in these essentially nonneurotic
types of disturbances can be taken to be the result or the
symptomatic expression of conflicts of a neurotic nature.
These manifestations are rather dependent on a set of etio-
logical factors that lead to deviations in development in one
or many areas of the personality and finally to "atypical development" and "atypical personalities." This is well illus-
trated, for example, in cases of institutionalized children in
whom the lack of what seems to constitute essential requirements (in terms of human contact and need of stimulation)
leads to distorted and retarded development of the personality and in the end to atypical personalities of a well-known
type. On the other hand, these cases show a great deal that is
"normal or nearly so," as well as many neurotic conflicts or
even more organized forms of neurosis. The latter can readily be understood on the basis of our psychoanalytic model
and for this reason it may be very tempting to interpret all
the other and no less relevant aspects of the disturbance as
arising from conflicts of a neurotic nature. The fact, however,
is that these are completely different phenomena, the genetic
roots of which can in some cases be found very early in life.

2 The title of another symposium held in 1954.

Only those authors who have lost sight of this basic distinction could regard this type of case as a neurosis—a generalization which is not justified. The genetic equation of all these disturbances is a simple step, but a mistaken one, I believe; yet it has unfortunately been taken by many. Perhaps the enthusiasm produced by the insights gained into these disturbances has at least temporarily obscured the fact that in spite of the similarities between many of these disturbances there also exist basic differences that must be accounted for.

Another factor obscuring some of the basic issues has resulted from the uneven growth of insight in psychoanalysis. Thus, the general position of the oedipus complex in every neurosis was clearly established in the late nineties, though the term itself was introduced somewhat later. The first analysis of a child (Little Hans) brought direct observations of the conflicts that had previously been reconstructed in the analysis of adults. Although at this time (1909) the concept of a developmental sequence leading to and influencing the infantile neurosis was well established in Freud's mind, really comprehensive formulations of the phases that precede and influence the "infantile neurosis" were put forward only later, in some cases many years later. It was only in 1913 that Freud described the anal phase (or rather the anal-sadistic stage) as well as its various contributions to personality development in terms of the vicissitudes of the different component instincts characteristic of that phase.[3] With these formulations Freud made an essential contribution to the problem of the choice of neurosis, a problem that had preoccupied Freud for many years. For the first time attention was called to the fact that important fixations at the anal stage played a significant role in the development of certain disturbances and especially in the development of the obsessional neurosis. The concept of the "oral phase" first appeared in the 1915 edition of *The Three Essays* (1905,

[3] See "The Disposition to Obsessional Neurosis" (1913a).

p. 197f.); with this it became possible to understand the contribution of the component instincts of this phase to personality development and to appreciate the importance of fixation points at this early stage for certain forms of psychopathology.

In terms of the theory of infantile neurosis it is of special significance that the "phallic phase" was conceptualized much later than the two earlier pregenital phases of development. The phallic phase as we understand it now was described only in 1923. At that time the oedipus complex was solidly anchored to this specific phase and its regular occurrence at the ages of two to five years firmly established. This is of course the time at which the infantile neurosis makes its appearance.

In this way the role of the oedipus complex and its corollary, the infantile neurosis, was overshadowed by the discovery of the pregenital phases and of their essential contributions to normal development and, even more important, to pathological development in the case of significant fixations at these pregenital stages. All these discoveries concentrated attention on these phases, especially perhaps on the oral phase at the expense of the others. Some analysts began to view these early phases as the only important stages in development and neglected the later phases that *especially in the case of neurosis* always play an essential role and make an essential contribution to the personality as a whole.

In her paper "Psychoanalysis and Education" (1954) Anna Freud pointed to the fact that of the many attempts to trace back the beginning of neurotic development to the earliest libidinal phase, i.e., the oral phase, little has reached the lay public beyond the misunderstood notion that only the behavior of the mother (an environmental factor) proves decisive for the child's mental health or illness. She concluded that: "To put the blame for the infantile neurosis on the mother's shortcoming in the oral phase is no more than a facile and misleading generalization. Analysis has to probe further and deeper in its search for the causation of neurosis" (p. 11).[4]

Much of the ensuing discussion at the symposium (see Kris et al., 1954) was an attempt to deal with this type of oversimplification and to point to the complexity of interaction of internal and external factors in development. Anna Freud, for example, commented on Waelder's helpful formulation "that the mother, as the earliest and foremost representative of the environment, has a selective influence upon the constitutional endowment by stimulating and encouraging some things and discouraging others" (p. 62). She herself has expressed the same view at different times. Anna Freud further stated: "By rejecting and seducing she [the mother] can influence, distort and determine development, but she cannot produce either neurosis or psychosis. I believe we ought to view the influence of the mother in this respect against the background of the spontaneous developmental forces which are active in the child. Then we are faced by the question how far innate trends toward the normal can be deflected by environmental influence" (p. 62). Both Anna Freud and Robert Waelder agreed that the answer to this problem is best served by Freud's approach of the "complemental series" of external and internal factors.[5] The latter seem to me to remain an essential consideration for the developmental approach.

Melanie Klein and her followers claim that the oedipus complex is already well in evidence during the oral phase and more specifically during what she describes as the "depres-

4 This paper was delivered by Anna Freud as the Freud Anniversary Lecture at the New York Academy of Medicine. It was further discussed at the symposium on "Problems of Infantile Neurosis" (Kris et al., 1954).

5 All participants, among them Anna Freud, Ernst Kris, Hartmann, Greenacre, Mittelmann, were in agreement concerning the basic assumptions outlined above and long familiar to psychoanalysts. Ernst Kris, for example, referred to the "variants in needs" of infants, to which Anna Freud commented, "I want to emphasize that I am, like himself, a firm believer in the constitutional differences between infants" (p. 60). Mittelmann pointed out that not all constitutional or congenital tendencies are manifest at birth but that some become operative at different points in development (p. 64).

sive position." Hanna Segal (1964) points out: "It is implicit
in Melanie Klein's definition of the depressive position that
the oedipus complex begins to develop during this phase, of
which it is an integral part" (p. 90).[6]

Hanna Segal describes the first part of the oral stage, last-
ing three to four months, as the "paranoid schizoid position."
The "depressive position" is placed in the second part of the
oral phase (during the second half of the first year of life).
Both "positions," viewed as subdivisions of the oral stage
(p. xii), are characterized by specific forms of object relations,
anxieties, and defenses. Problems met at later stages, including the "genital form" of the oedipus complex, "can be
tackled within a paranoid-schizoid or a depressive pattern"
(p. xiii).

In short, according to Melanie Klein, the whole personality evolves from the "paranoid-schizoid and depressive positions" as experienced during the first year of life. With the
relative working through of the depressive position that has
superseded the paranoid and schizoid position, neurotic
mechanisms take over from the psychotic one; finally, repara-
tion, sublimation, and creativity tend to replace both the
neurotic and the more primitive psychotic mechanisms.

In Melanie Klein's view, the "infantile neurosis" and
apparently the "phallic phase" as well are considered to be
"defensive structures." In Hanna Segal's words: "Thus, in
Melanie Klein's view, infantile neurosis is a defence against
underlying paranoid and depressive anxieties, and a way of
binding and working them through" (p. xiii). And: "It will
be clear from what I have said so far that in Melanie Klein's
view, the child has an awareness of both the male and female
genital from quite early on and that the phallic phase and the

6 These views can be assumed to be representative of the Kleinian formulations since they are taken from a book based on a series of lectures given for
years at the London Institute of Psycho-Analysis by one of the leading Kleinian analysts, as an introduction for students of psychoanalysis to Melanie
Klein's work.

phantasy of the phallic woman are defensive structures—one of the versions of the combined parents" (p. 95).

Although these views are for the most part not acceptable to the large majority of analysts, there can be no doubt that this type of formulation has played an important role in the dilution and obscurity of the concept of the "infantile neurosis" as originally formulated by Freud and further elaborated by many other analysts.

The fact that certain events taking place during the oral stages, or rather during the first year of life, can shape the personality in what seem to be irreversible and undesirable outcomes (an extreme example of it can be seen in the cases of institutionalized children described above) should not distract us from the equally important fact that health or neurotic emotional disturbances in childhood as well as in adults depend on the appropriate resolution of the oedipus complex and the infantile neurosis.

CHAPTER 3

DEVELOPMENTAL INTERFERENCE

A "developmental interference" can be defined as whatever disturbs the typical unfolding of development. The term may be reserved to describe those situations that involve gross external (environmental) interference with certain needs and rights of the child or situations in which unjustified demands are made of the child. In making such demands the environment frequently does not take into account the child's lack of ego capacity to comply or cope with them. The disturbance thus introduced may sometimes affect development in positive ways but usually affects it in negative ways.

It must be added that many developmental interferences are not meant to happen. They can be described as accidental, as in cases of long separations of mother and child due to prolonged illness or hospitalization of the mother.

In another group of cases the interference is culturally determined and actively imposed on the child by society through its representatives, the mother or other figures in authority. To cite but two examples: early and rigidly imposed toilet training; feeding on a fixed, inflexible timetable of four hours apart, with no regard for individual needs and variations.

The cases referred to so far cover those situations where something is done to the infant or to the child either in an active manner or accidentally by the environment or its

28

representatives. No less significant is the case where the developmental interference comes about, not through excessive, inappropriate, and nonage-adequate stimulation or demands, but through the lack of the indispensable minimum of stimulation and interaction between the baby and his mother or his environment.

It is well established that the healthy development of the infant requires these interactions and that their lack alters the normal unfolding of the developmental processes, leading to retardations and distortions that can under specific circumstances become irreversible.[1] Thus the lack of provision of these stimulations constitutes a gross "interference" with what are the *sine qua non* requirements for the unfolding of normal development.

The degree to which certain types of interference will influence the child clearly depends on their nature and on the specific developmental stage at which they occur. While some interferences with the child's needs or developmental rights are essentially phase-specific, the impact of others will differ with the child's age. It is not possible to give an exhaustive account of all the possible forms of developmental interferences at the different stages in the child's life. I shall limit myself to the enumeration of a small number of situations which occur very frequently and which are representative examples.

One such interference is the separation of the child from the mother at a time when the child has a strong biological need for and right to the mother's presence. Enforced separations due to parental holidays, hospitalizations, and other reasons will lead to upheavals in the emotional life of the child, upheavals with which he cannot cope with the resources at his disposal. Another such interference is observed in cases of marked and prolonged depression of the mother at the beginning of the child's life. Further possible interfer-

[1] See the work of Anna Freud, René Spitz, and more recently the outstanding work of Provence and Lipton in their book *Infants in Institutions* (1962).

ences are exposure to hunger through neglect or rigid feeding time tables; hospitalization of the child (a factor which can act as an interference either because of the separation or because of traumatic medical manipulations); illness of a painful nature and of prolonged duration; surgical interventions such as tonsillectomy or appendectomy taking place during the phallic-oedipal phase may act as a trigger for certain forms of the infantile neurosis; very early or rigid toilet training; death of parents, siblings, or other important persons (the points at which these experiences occur in the child's life being particularly significant for his later development).

The following two examples may help to illustrate some of the points made:

CASE 1

C. S. was three years four months old at the time of referral. Her mother brought her to the Clinic because she wanted advice about nursery schools and because of a skin irritation of a year's duration, said to have started the day after the father permanently left home. For this reason the mother was convinced that its cause was psychological.

Mrs. S. was a trained nursery school teacher, who now worked as an artist and sculptor. She was very anxious for the child to develop well emotionally. Her marriage had been a bad one from the time when the child was two months old; the father finally left the home a few months before referral and the mother was now trying to obtain a divorce from him. She maintained that her husband, a teacher in a school for delinquent children, was addicted to marijuana.

The child's early history was characterized by the following significant events. At about two months C. was weaned to the bottle so that she could be placed in a day nursery; the reason for this was that the marriage was not going well, the parents having agreed to separate, and the mother was looking for a job. At about four months C. was placed in a day nursery until the age of eight months when the parents tried to resume the marriage. During the first week of the placement at the day nursery C. refused many of the feedings and developed severe diarrhea. After this she began to feed normally at the nursery. This was the first of a series of separations from the mother to which C. reacted with a number of disturbances.

C. then stayed home with her mother for five months, that is, from eight to thirteen months. Unfortunately during this time Mrs. S. became pregnant and had a miscarriage. At this point C. was taken to her maternal aunt for a stay of three weeks. The mother believed that the child had been upset by this separation. Since that time C. has been anxious about losing her mother and has clung to her.

Between the ages of one to two and a half C. had been sent to nursery school; however, because the mother never found them to be satisfactory, there had been several changes of schools. At the time of referral the mother was again looking for another nursery school so that she could get on with her work; for this reason she was intent on finding an all-day nursery.

When C. was two years and nine months old, Mrs. S. went to the hospital for gynecological treatment. This time C. went to stay with a friend of Mrs. S., a woman who had two little boys about C.'s age. As the result of this separation C. started to wet the bed every night. She had previously been dry at night since the age of two years. She also developed a sleep disturbance (to which other factors not discussed here probably have contributed). Whereas she had always slept well at night and in her own room, she now often wanted to sleep with her mother and to cuddle with her in what the mother felt was a very sensual way.

C. was described as a very alert, intelligent, and highly verbal little girl. Her physical development had always tended to be somewhat slow and she still was rather small for her age. She liked best to have her mother around. As long as she knew that the mother was at home C. was quite content to go out and play, e.g., in the garden with other children, but she would keep looking up to make sure her mother was in the studio which C. could see from the garden. The child was very attached to the mother and hated to leave her.

There was a new threat hanging over the child: the mother talked of sending C. abroad to her grandparents in the near future, although she apparently had not yet made a final decision.

It was clear that the child because of the many separations since early in life suffered from "true separation anxiety." This was shown in the regression, symptoms, and psychosomatic disturbances which C. developed during such periods. A very illustrative example took place during the psychiatric interview. It shows clearly how pressing the mother's own needs and fears were and how, partly because of this, she overlooked, denied, or distorted realities concerning the child's well-being.

Mrs. S. wanted to talk privately with the psychiatrist interviewing C. The psychiatrist replied that this would be rather difficult because C. should not be left alone in the waiting room; however, he would try to arrange a special appointment with her. After proposing several unsuitable solutions, she said, "We will have to make the best of it," and then told C. to go downstairs and wait for her in "that room we were in before." The psychiatrist could not believe that she was going to send the child downstairs by herself and thought that he had misheard, but in a second she opened the door, half-pushed the child through it, closed the door behind the child, saying, "She is a very independent child." The psychiatrist went outside where C. was standing looking bewildered and ready to cry. When she saw the mother through the open door, C. went back into the room and said to her mother, "You come with me." The psychiatrist then insisted that Mrs. S. take the child down to the waiting room and that he could talk with her only if C. was prepared to wait for a few minutes and if there was an adult to look after C.; otherwise it would be better to make another appointment.

Mrs. S. took C. downstairs and returned immediately, saying: "She'll be all right, she's got a jigsaw. Now about this I.Q. . . ." A few seconds later the sound of a child crying in distress became audible in the room. When the psychiatrist wondered whether that was C., the mother listened for a moment, concluded that it was not C., and attempted to proceed with her interrogation. The psychiatrist thought it would be better to go out and check. He found C. crying bitterly on the floor above. When they met, Mrs. S. said: "So it was her, my, my, what's all the crying about?" C. sobbed that she could not find her mummy.

Summary of Salient Events and C.'s Reaction to Them

At four months, placement in a day nursery: C. developed gastrointestinal disturbances in the form of severe diarrhea and food refusal.

At eight to thirteen months, mother's pregnancy and miscarriage, followed by C.'s three-week stay with maternal aunt: C. was upset and began to be anxious about losing the mother; started to cling to her.

When C. was first sent to nursery school, she developed several colds.

At two years and nine months (mother in the hospital for gynecological treatment) C. went to a friend: C. reacted with regression to bed wetting, sleep disturbance, increased clinging and anxiety about losing mother.

Shortly thereafter the father left home permanently: C.'s skin irritation is said to have started the day after the father left.

This child, it must be noted, has a good ego, which has helped her a great deal to cope with all the "separations" from her mother. This is clearly seen as well in her ability to settle down—at a very early age after an initial period of upset—in nursery school; moreover, she had to cope with the added complication of the many changes of nursery school, frequently implying adaptation to a new surrounding and new objects (children and adults). C. was able to participate in the activities at the nursery and to become interested in the material and equipment provided. She was also able to form close friendships with some of the children.

While the various interferences with some of the child's basic needs have not hindered her in achieving many age-adequate developmental tasks, the amount and degree of interference led to the disturbances described above. The picture was further complicated by the existence of other forms of interference which, for the sake of simplicity, I have not discussed here; these relate to her phallic-oedipal position and identifications. Apart from the disturbances described, other factors will influence her further personality development: there are the contributions resulting from these age-specific interferences and the existence of a set of circumstances which in her later life may lead to undesirable identifications.

CASE 2

A. B., two years one month old, was brought to the Hampstead Clinic because of feeding difficulties that had started at age one year. Until that time she had eaten very well. She then began to refuse to feed herself and instead ran around the table and played; she could be induced to eat only with much coaxing or by giving her toys.

While she previously had been a very good sleeper, she developed a sleep disturbance three months before referral.

Mrs. B. connected the eating difficulty with an episode of enteritis when A. was one year old. A. lost her appetite and was in a very poor condition for two to three weeks. However, Mrs. B. believed that A.'s reluctance to eat had actually started earlier than the enteritis episode: somewhere around the time when the child was ten months old and the mother's second pregnancy began. Mrs. B. also believed that the eating problem has become even more difficult since the birth of A.'s sister. At that time when A. was nineteen months old, she spent four weeks with the maternal grandmother while the mother was in the hospital. After A.'s return home, she frequently did not want to eat.

The sleeping problem developed recently when the parents moved to a new house. Because of the move and during it A. was again sent to the maternal grandmother for a week. There she was put to sleep for the first time in a small bed instead of a cot.

On her return home A. went back to sleep in her cot but started screaming when the mother left her. Mrs. B. wondered whether the child was afraid of the dark or the strangeness of the new house and left the door open for her. A. seemed happy and went off to sleep.

Unfortunately three weeks later the mother decided to move A. to a new bed and to let A.'s younger sister have A.'s cot. (It should be added here that A. showed many signs of strong jealousy of the sister which the mother was forced to deny completely.) In a few days A. began waking up and crying. If the mother did not come to her, A. would go and curl up on the floor outside the parents' bedroom door, going back and forth from her room to theirs. As a result of all this, A. was tired during the day and the mother was affected as well.

Comment

It will have been noticed that this was a mother full of good intention, but not always in touch with the child's needs. She frequently overlooked what the child reacted to and had no awareness of the effect of the separations, birth of the sister, change of bed, jealousy of the sister—events which this child was forced to cope with in quick succession.

Like C., the little girl of the first example, A. tried very hard to comply with the demands made on her, but for such a young child the demands were far too many and spaced in a very short period of time.

Clearly, the same type of interference may produce different results and reactions in different children. Although it is possible to discern some general tendencies depending on the type of interference and the age of the child, each case must be assessed individually. Different backgrounds, different previous experiences, different internal circumstances may either reinforce or soften the effect of a given interference.

As can be seen from the examples referred to, children react to the upheavals created by the developmental interferences with abnormal manifestations which in many instances greatly resemble those observed in the case of neurotic conflict or neurosis proper; that is, they react with anxiety, multiple forms of regression on the side of the drives, occasionally by giving up certain ego achievements, and by developing abnormal forms of behavior.

This group of "symptoms" is on the surface identical with those symptoms that result from compromise formations in neurotic conflicts. Closer examination, however, shows that there are important metapsychological differences between these symptoms. The "symptoms" occurring early in life are frequently not compromise formations with symbolic unconscious meaning and content (the symptom itself implying a certain amount of indirect unconscious gratification); rather, they are specific reactions and are devoid of any of the advantages that a conflict solution by means of compromise formation in the form of symptoms achieves. On the other hand, as the child grows older, the developmental interference will be interpreted in terms of the developmental stage through which the child is going. A traumatic surgical intervention at the peak of the phallic-oedipal phase may be interpreted as a punishment for his oedipal strivings and masturbation fantasies. In this case the interference acts by greatly reinforcing and increasing the intensity and difficulties of what is otherwise a normal phase in the development of the child, with its typical developmental conflict, that is, the phallic-oedipal conflict. In this way the fate of his phallic organization may be determined along lines which are not the most desirable.

It is important to re-emphasize that the impact of developmental interferences on the child's future development varies greatly with the age of the child, the level of ego and drive development at the time of the interference, as well as with other factors. While not all developmental interferences automatically damage the structure of the personality, I think there can be little doubt that many personalities are decisively shaped by such interferences, especially if they occur at crucial developmental phases and are operative for a prolonged period of time. We know that ego development is in part determined by interactions between the child's inner potentialities and his environment. If certain forms of interference affecting specific ego functions occur sufficiently early in life, the ego may take on a different shape. Such occurrences may in fact account for individual variations in functioning and for the wide range of variations of normality.

The very same considerations, however, also pose the interesting problem that some of the results of these interferences (in terms of personality development) may be neither reversible nor accessible to psychoanalytic technique. For example, the provision of stimulation at a later stage cannot redirect development that was stunted as a result of the lack of care required in babyhood.

Furthermore, these early disturbances, these developmental interferences, when they are of a detrimental nature, will determine the outcome of subsequent developmental conflicts, neurotic conflicts, the infantile neurosis, and the neurosis of adulthood. They may lead, for example, through excessive frustration or even excessive gratification, to the establishment of important fixation points at one or more levels. Thus, when the child is later confronted by the usual developmental conflicts—especially by those characteristic of the phallic-oedipal phase—he may not be capable of mastering them satisfactorily. With much of his libido and aggression remaining behind at early fixation points, he may not have available sufficient amounts of libido and aggression capable of forward movements. Thus, a firm position cannot be established at later developmental stages and the usual phase-specific conflicts may prove too strong for his weak drive organization. No less important is the constant pull backwards exerted by these early fixation points. A combination of factors such as these may bring about a collapse of the personality when the individual is confronted by conflicts or other stresses, either in childhood or adulthood.

Clearly, then, the developmental interferences will in different ways make contributions to the process of structuralization of the different aspects of the personality. This accounts for both the many variations of normality and certain abnormal and undesirable character traits. As mentioned above, they also lay the ground on which later neurotic conflicts will develop. Moreover, they largely determine the type of conflict that may develop, its forms of expression, and its severity.

Precisely because the developmental interferences can have such a variety of effects, it is important to study the specific factors operative in each case. As we learn more about what influences development in positive or negative ways, it will be possible to avoid harmful manipulations, demands, and expectations in favor of those whose beneficial effect is recognized. As a result preventive intervention can be more effective.

Finally, I want to point out that the adult too can be subjected to massive interference by stresses or life situations which greatly resemble those I have described for the child. Their influence, however, is of a very different nature because the adult personality structure is fully developed. It can no longer be patterned according to these interferences as was possible in the case of the child. Furthermore, the adult is much better equipped to cope with stresses for the very reason that he is a finished product; he has a fully developed ego and superego, can choose among several alternatives of coping as well as multiple forms of drive gratification. Nevertheless, some of these interferences in later life may act as the triggering situation upsetting the inner balance and economy. With the loss of equilibrium a previously latent neurosis may move to the foreground. In other cases the "abnormal reaction" will disappear or recede as soon as the "massive (traumatic) interference" is no longer present. Persons in the first group presumably have a personality structure in which the balance of forces is more unstable and which contains tendencies favorable for the development of neurotic conflicts when the precarious inner equilibrium is lost. Persons in the second group presumably possess a basically more healthy structure which enables them to recover as soon as the traumatic conditions are removed. To disturb their equilibrium, therefore, requires a far greater amount of interference than in the first group. Yet, in view of the fact that each adult has an individual history and was exposed to specific early interferences that shaped his character, proclivities, and vulnerabilities, the impact of interferences in his adult life will therefore depend not only on their intensity but also on their specific nature.

Returning once more to the child, it must be noted that most developmental interferences are of the nature of conflicts between the child's drives and his environment. Anna Freud (1962) has described them as "external conflicts,"[2] in contrast to "internalized conflicts" which are conflicts between the different structures (id, ego, superego), once the originally external conflicts have become part of the intrapsychic structure and act as the inner representative of the external world. "Internalized conflicts" must be distinguished as well from the "internal conflicts" (ambivalence, bisexuality, etc.) typical of human nature.

[2] See also Nagera (1963).

I also wish to emphasize that such conflicts with the external world when they act as developmental interferences do not always manifest themselves in symptom formation or disorders of behavior. Instead of leading to symptom formation, they frequently favor certain forms of structuralization or make a contribution to the development of certain character traits through internalization of the external demands or through identification with the external authority.

CHAPTER 4

DEVELOPMENTAL CONFLICTS

"Developmental Conflicts" are experienced by every child to a greater or lesser degree either when certain specific environmental demands are made at the appropriate developmental phases, or when the child reaches certain developmental and maturational levels at which specific conflicts are created. Toilet training demanded at the appropriate time and in a reasonable form is an example of what is meant in the first case, while the developments observed at the time of the phallic-oedipal phase illustrate the second instance. Most frequently a combination of both factors is involved.

Occasionally, what should have been one of the usual developmental conflicts can be transformed as well into a very serious developmental interference when the demand, even if correct in timing, is made in improper or even traumatic ways, that is, when there is a gross interference with the child's rights and needs on the side of the environment.[1]

If we elaborate further our hypothetical example concerning toilet training, it is clear that a specific degree of maturation of the central nervous system (myelinization of the pyramidal tracts, etc.) must have occurred before voluntary sphincter control is at all feasible. Nevertheless, "training" can also be effected by circumventing conscious control by means of reflex conditioning, long before the child is ready

[1] Individual variations have to be taken into consideration and for this purpose age alone is insufficient. As is well known, under normal conditions the rate of development varies greatly among different children. Both physical and emotional readiness is required before the specific demands are put forward by the mother or the environment.

41

(physically or maturationally) and before he can understand, accept, and comply with such requirements. Not infrequently such attempts at early training have harmful consequences, some of which could be considered to be serious developmental interferences (see Chapter 3). For example, the child may be forced to sit on a pot for hours at a time when this restriction of his motility is least welcome. The child frequently reacts violently to this unjustified demand, and serious battles ensue with an unhappy, annoyed, shouting, and in extreme cases punishing mother. The developmental interference here is related to the restriction of motility and the negative aspects of the mother-child relationship.

In any case at some point this child will move to the anal phase and begin to cathect and highly value his body products. Furthermore, at about the same time he will begin to develop concern for the feelings and wishes of the object. Thus the external demand for cleanliness made in this period finds an echo in the internal structure of the child. He values his feces highly, but now he values as much and even more the mother who demands that he renounce his anal pleasures. Clearly, it is somewhere at this stage that the child is ready to comply with the environmental demands for cleanliness if they are presented to him with understanding and awareness of his conflicting wishes. Readiness thus implies his having reached the required physical maturity, the appropriate phase of instinctual development, the necessary ego development, and the corresponding stage of object relationships.

In this sequence we can observe how what was previously a gross developmental interference[2] has become a true develop-

[2] Note that previously the interference did not necessarily involve the child's anal instinctual drives to start with, but rather involved a restriction of his motility. In any case, before and at the beginning of his anal phase the child's instinctual wish is quite clear and straightforward. He has no conflict as yet within himself on account of the gratification of some of his anal component instincts. The conflict is with the outside world that demands performance in specific places, at regular intervals, and so forth.

mental conflict through growth, maturation, and developmental processes taking place in the child. This could also be referred to as an "internal developmental conflict" because there are now two opposite tendencies "inside the child himself," one a representative of his drives or id tendencies, the other an internal representative of the previously external demands in the form of early superego precursors.

When the internalization of the external demands has been more or less fully accomplished, this specific developmental conflict disappears, because the balance has plainly shifted from the need to gratify the instinctual demands to the need to comply with the now internal representatives of the external demands. A further step toward structuralization and character formation has thus been taken as the result of the solution of a developmental conflict. This achievement comes about only slowly and gradually, proceeding via a series that starts at one end with a minimum of conflict (due to the limited internalization) and having at the other extreme full internalization. Thus the developmental conflicts may start at one end of the scale as an admixture of different elements of "external" and "internalized" conflicts, while at the other end they are fully internalized.

There is no doubt that the existence of gross developmental interference—at an early age and in areas which in due time are bound to produce one of the typical developmental conflicts—must contribute to shape these developmental conflicts and influence their outcome in a negative way.

It is well known that some phallic activity (though not phallic dominance) is observed very early in childhood. Children's masturbatory activity can begin long before the phallic phase and can be met by an intolerant environment with all sorts of threats and actual punishment. Nevertheless, these threats usually become fully operative only when the child's development proceeds to the phallic phase. At this stage the penis receives an extremely large and intense cathexis that turns this organ into the most valuable possession. It is for this reason that the ego awareness of the existence of penisless objects becomes acute. All the previous observations the child made in this connection—and they did not disturb him too much then—now become fully meaningful and terrifying.[3] Similar observations in this phase provoke massive castration anxiety and fully confirm his now very intense castration fears. His oedipal love for the mother and his hate (and love) of the rival father now bring to the fore in full intensity the most important of all the possible developmental conflicts, that is, the oedipus conflict.

Excessive or traumatic interference with the child's masturbation before the phallic-oedipal phase can be described as a developmental interference. By the time the child reaches the phallic-oedipal phase this developmental interference has been transformed into a developmental conflict because of the maturational steps that have taken place in the ego, on the side of the drives, and in the sphere of object relationships.

At this point it is convenient to call attention to the danger of placing too much emphasis on external circumstances as the triggering factor of many neurotic episodes in childhood. This is frequently done without paying due attention or giving sufficient consideration to the internal changes constantly taking place in the child as the result of the ongoing maturational and developmental processes. In fact, it is frequently these inner changes that make certain environmental happenings into meaningful and traumatic episodes capable of triggering a neurotic development or creating the necessary background for such disturbances.

It is not possible to give an account of all the possible developmental conflicts. A number of them, such as the two cited above, are very common and typical in the development

3 This shows the degree to which a young child's ego awareness is linked with and partially dependent on where his drive interests are. For a child in the oral phase the world is an oral world, largely understood in oral terms. Similarly in the anal and phallic phases, many external events are interpreted with reference to the phase-dominant drive concerns.

of all children. On the other hand, I am inclined to assume that different children may have—apart from the common traditional ones—some specific and individual developmental conflicts that are based on an interaction between strong innate tendencies of specific component instincts and an environment which strongly objects to them. The individual nature of such conflicts is due to the fact that the intensity of the different component instincts varies greatly from one child to another, as do the environmental reactions to them. The "environment" is after all composed of highly individual parents, each having his own unique characteristics.

The developmental conflicts are usually phase specific and of a transitory nature. In normal circumstances they generally disappear more or less completely once a specific phase has passed and further forward developmental moves have occurred. While these developmental conflicts are active we may observe anxiety of different types, some temporary symptom formation, some behavioral disorders, some phase-specific fears. As mentioned before, the developmental conflict may be swept away by the next wave of developmental progression or at least largely recede into the background as a result of it.

An example based on observations of one child in our nursery shows how one developmental conflict solved itself normally as soon as the particular phase creating it was left behind. The conflict concerned some of the anal impulses of the child. Before describing these observations, two nursery school children are compared in this respect. Both boys were two and a half years old at the time of these observations.

S.'s friend, G., at this stage showed his obsessional character, safeguarding himself by means of ever-changing rituals. S., too, had rituals at this time, but they never lasted very long and were not replaced by others when they were given up, e.g., the *brown* smarties [chocolate sweets coated with sugar in different colors] or the white woollen cap (that he used for several days), the tidy clothes and a special movement with his shoulders as if to ward off a fly which bothered him.[4]

At snack time the children had smarties. When S. (aged two and a half) still had about four of them left on his plate, he asked for some more. But the teacher told him that he should first finish those on his plate. S. did not reply to this, but neither did he eat his smarties, all of which were brown. The teacher then put another handful on S.'s plate, and he again ate all colors except the brown ones.

A month later, at snack time the children again had smarties. When the teacher came to S., he expressly requested not to be given any brown ones. On past Tuesdays when he got smarties he always left the brown ones untouched on his plate, saying, when asked, that he didn't like them.

Two months later (S. was two years nine months) we had smarties at snack time. Whereas in the past S. always left all brown smarties untouched, he ate them today like the others. He was quite aware of what he was doing and did not eat them by accident. This became obvious when the teacher asked him about his eating the brown smarties now and he said that he did not mind them any more and liked them now just like the others.[5]

In some cases the solution of the developmental conflict is achieved through certain specific steps in structuralization. Some modified forms of drive expression, or of reaction formations and sublimations of the specific component instincts, are incorporated into the personality in the shape of character traits. In this way oral, anal, and phallic characters, or combinations of them in various degrees of intensity, come about.

In still other cases either unfavorable circumstances or the intensity of the developmental conflict may lead to the establishment of important fixation points. These will not only influence the child's further development in general[6] but

---

4 Report to the Educational Unit, May, 1964, by Mrs. M. Friedman, the nursery school head-teacher at the Hampstead Clinic.

5 These observations of the Afternoon Group were recorded by A. Holder.

6 In this respect it must be borne in mind that the younger child is both much more vulnerable to and malleable by conflicts occurring in early life.

create favorable conditions for later disturbances, in a way very similar to that described for the developmental interferences.

In order to cope with developmental conflicts the ego may put forward specific defense mechanisms, the effects of which deserve closer examination. On the one hand, the use of some defenses may interfere with the appropriate performance of specific ego functions. Observation and research in this area will determine in which ways a child's development (on the ego side or otherwise) is affected when, early in life, it has to proceed without recourse to a number of normally available ego functions. The same applies in cases of early neurotic conflicts.

In the adult the impact of defense activity in case of neurosis or neurotic conflicts will produce a similar type of interference with one or another ego function. However, since the development of the adult is completed, the impact can no longer shape development as it can in the case of the child.

I have referred to the differences between developmental interferences and developmental conflicts and at the same time emphasized the possibility of a continuum in many cases. Thus certain developmental interferences can in due time become developmental conflicts, and their mishandling will add to certain developmental conflicts the characteristics and qualities of the developmental interferences. In the following chapters I shall highlight the similarities, differences, and relationships between developmental conflicts and neurotic conflicts and then the similarities, differences, and relationships between developmental conflicts, the infantile neurosis, and the neurosis of adulthood.

CHAPTER 5

NEUROTIC CONFLICTS

This term as it is usually employed in psychoanalysis and general psychiatry has many connotations. Here I shall restrict its meaning to conflicts that take place among the different psychic structures, id, ego, and the superego; the latter either as a final structure or in early childhood more frequently its precursors, long before the establishment of the final superego structure. The "neurotic conflicts" are simple units. They result from component instincts pushing for gratification and other aspects of the personality opposing such gratification, that is, forces in the form of internalized demands (representing the external prohibition). Neurotic conflicts can occur very early in the life of infants. We distinguish them from "neurosis proper," which has a much more complex organization and as such appears only at a much later stage in the child's development. The neurosis proper can and usually does include several neurotic conflicts. We also distinguish neurotic conflicts from conflicts between the child's drives and the external world[1] by the fact that the objection to the discharge or the gratification is in the case of the neurotic conflicts an internalized one.

Neurotic conflicts frequently are remnants of previous developmental conflicts. Typically, developmental conflicts are specific of certain phases or stages in development. Under

[1] External conflicts in the Developmental Profile (see Anna Freud, 1962, 1965; and Nagera, 1963).

48

ideal conditions they should disappear as soon as the next stage is reached, partly because a shift in the energy distribution occurs with each new developmental move. Moving into the foreground, a new group of component instincts acquires full force, while the group of previously dominant component instincts recedes into the background. From then onward they make no more than the normal contribution to the dynamics of the personality, and the conflict disappears.

In cases where the strength of the component instincts involved in the conflict is greater, due to individual variations, the developmental conflict may be solved in such a way that some aspects of the component instincts objected to are taken into the personality in the form of character traits. Such component instincts may be taken in either directly (with some displacement and aim inhibitions) or as reaction formations against them. However, some developmental conflicts cannot be solved in this manner and when development proceeds further, they remain behind as unresolved conflictive areas. In this way what should have been a transitory developmental conflict becomes a permanent neurotic conflict. Thus it should be noted that a neurotic conflict is frequently the continuation of a developmental conflict that has not resolved itself properly at the appropriate time. Some developmental conflicts could be described as "transitory neurotic conflicts" or still better as *"transitory developmental neurotic conflicts."* Transitory conflicts are thus turned into permanent conflictive areas with permanent pockets of anxiety or symptom formation of a restricted nature.

As in the case of developmental interferences and of developmental conflicts, the neurotic conflicts will make a contribution to the further development of the personality, including its conflict-free and autonomous aspects. Once an ego function, for example, attention, is caught in the neurotic conflict and is affected, then other related functions (memory, thinking, etc.) are also likely to show interference. The tendency to withdraw into fantasy as a defense against some

unpleasant aspects of reality will eventually affect the subject's perception of external reality as well as his memory.
Attention and concentration may similarly be involved. If
certain interferences take place when the child is very young,
for example, two years of age, his perceptual processes may
well be affected, and this may pave the way for later pre-
ferred ways of assimilating information (visually or audito-
rily). The neurotic conflicts create favorable conditions for the
subsequent development of more complex and organized
forms of neurosis. The impact of neurotic conflicts will vary,
depending on how long they have remained active, what
drives are involved, and how strong and significant these are
in any given personality.

The fate of neurotic conflicts, which may occur at any
point in the child's development, varies greatly. Some of them
will remain active and integrate themselves into the infantile
neuroses (which, on the other hand, they have helped to
shape) and at a later stage into the adolescent or the adulthood neurosis. Others will remain active for some time and
then, partly because of the increase in ego strength and the
new abilities that maturation has contributed, they may suc-
cumb to the now stronger and more efficient defense activity.[2]

Since neurotic conflicts have been defined as conflicts of an
internalized nature, it may be appropriate to clarify the role
played by the superego and the superego precursors. It is
usually assumed that the final superego structure comes into
being only after the resolution of the oedipus conflict. It is
further assumed that at this point the superego acquires the
strength necessary for enforcing its demands. However, superego precursors begin to appear much earlier. I take the view
that very early processes of identification imply the presence
of introjects active as superego precursors. I further take the
view that some of the early introjections include not only a

---

[2] The type of defense used is in itself significant, because some defenses are
more favorable than others in terms of development and possibilities of ego
performance.

given prohibition or command but also the capacity to enforce them, that is, the necessary authority to see them through. For example, when toilet training is finally achieved and becomes an internal concern of the child himself, he is quite capable of enforcing and maintaining the achievement, independent of the presence or absence of the external authority that originally made the demand. The introjection carries with it the energy necessary to impose—*in so far as this type of impulse is concerned*—the required restrictions. We have observed in a number of our children a marked inhibition of oral aggression, starting late in the second half of the first year of life. In all these cases we have observed as well that their environment in general, and especially the mother, has evident conflicts with the expression of aggression and in some cases with oral-aggressive manifestations in particular.

CASE 3

A. S., now two and a half years old, had shown since she was about nine months old an inhibition of oral aggression, especially observable in relation to her inability to chew. The social history contained many hints about the mother's unconscious attitude toward oral aggression, most noticeable in the many references to the mother's need to wean the child as soon as she "started to teeth." This is very relevant in view of the child's present inability to chew and of her phobic attitude toward dogs, which is presumably based on the projection onto the dog of her now inhibited wish to bite.

There is further evidence that Mrs. S. is in conflict about the expression of aggression in any form. This can be seen, for example, in her attitude in relation to the now "phallic-aggressive" behavior of A.'s brother.

A.'s inhibition of chewing started quite early in her life and has persisted until the present day as a remnant of a neurotic conflict. It has been further elaborated and has acquired new forms of expression, as in the dog phobia and in some other slight symptoms recently developed.

Obviously, in these very early forms of neurotic conflict the ego is far from the developed organization it will become at a later stage. Nevertheless, some part aspects of it can be operative, even though in somewhat primitive ways, and create the type of conflict described.

The example that follows illustrates the persistence of neurotic conflicts as a result of the faulty solution of some typical developmental conflicts of the anal phase. The strong opposition of a young ego to the anal impulses created a situation of marked conflict and symptom formation on the basis of typical obsessional mechanisms.

CASE 4

I. S. was eleven years old when she came for diagnostic assessment to the Hampstead Clinic. She was described as having been an "excessively dirty baby," playing and smearing herself with feces. By the time she was two years old she was very upset when she was dirty and washed her hands a great deal. She had in fact what amounted to a washing compulsion at this very early age, a symptomatic behavior pointing to the severity of the "neurotic conflict," that is, the conflict between her anal component instincts and her ego. At this time she became dry and clean during the day, but bed wetting at night has never stopped. At the time of her referral she showed some rituallike pieces of behavior when she put her dolls to bed in her mother's room.

In the case of A. S. mentioned above, an even earlier situation of neurotic conflict was observed concerning the oral-aggressive component instincts. Thus it seems possible to speak of a superego, or rather a precursor, which is built up first around the oral component instincts, especially when they are particularly intense, followed by a superego precursor dealing with different aspects of the anal component instincts, and finally a superego precursor built around the phallic-oedipal drives. Obviously there are marked differences among different people as to the relative importance of the oral, anal, or phallic-oedipal elements in the final superego structure. This is partly due to the contribution of the different component instincts in different people. The stronger they are the more important is the contribution they make to the personality and to the processes of structuralization (including superego formation).

The resolution of the oedipus complex nevertheless remains the most important element in superego development. In relation to it, the superego structure will take its final shape.

I believe that some minor or encapsulated symptoms that affect only limited aspects of some patient's personality may well be the result of compromise formations derived from a restricted situation of conflict, such as the one described as neurotic conflict. Such symptoms may have been acquired quite early and persisted in a relatively unchanged form, while otherwise development proceeded satisfactorily and led to a well-structured personality with excellent functional capacities. We do not yet know much about the economic and dynamic conditions under which such useful adaptive outcomes take place, nor do we know why in some cases the same type of early neurotic conflicts will lead to further disturbances and finally to neurosis. The study of these economic and dynamic conditions is certainly a most promising area.

The cases described above should be distinguished from certain types of neurosis in which a great deal of conflict has been, as it were, encapsulated and condensed within a limited symptom area, so that at the cost of a minor inhibition, good performance and balance were achieved elsewhere. Anna Freud at the Hampstead Clinic has called our attention to the question of the economic value of symptom formation.[3] She has suggested that one should assess against each other the price of upkeep versus gain in all processes of defense and symptom formation.

3 Personal communication.

CHAPTER 6

THE INFANTILE NEUROSIS

Infantile neurosis is Freud's term for the disturbances and stresses that he considered to be the common fate of all human beings when they pass through the phallic-oedipal phase of development. He said: ". . . the neuroses of childhood are in the nature of regular episodes in a child's development" (1926a, p. 148). "We know that a human child cannot successfully complete its development . . . without passing through a phase of neurosis sometimes of greater and sometimes of less distinctness" (1927, p. 42). "It has been found to be characteristic of a normal individual that he learns to master his Oedipus complex, whereas the neurotic subject remains involved in it" (1923, pp. 245-246).

He stated explicitly on several occasions that the oedipus complex is the "nuclear complex" of neurosis. Thus, he said: "It is to be suspected that, together with its extensions, it constitutes the *nuclear complex* of every neurosis, and we may expect to find it no less actively at work in other regions of mental life" (1910, p. 47). And: ". . . infantile sexuality, which is held under repression, acts as the chief motive force in the formation of symptoms; and the essential part of its content, the Oedipus complex, is the nuclear complex of neuroses" (1919, p. 204).

Little Hans, as is well known, was the first case of "infantile neurosis" ever treated by the psychoanalytic method.

54

Freud described the special value for him of this case as follows: "Strictly speaking, I learnt nothing . . . that I had not already been able to discover (though often less distinctly and more indirectly) from other patients analysed at a more advanced age. But the neuroses of these other patients could in every instance be traced back to the same infantile complexes that were revealed behind Hans's phobia. I am, therefore, tempted to claim for this neurosis of childhood the significance of being a type and a model" (1909, p. 147). A similar statement appears in the posthumously published *Outline:* "It seems that neuroses are acquired only in early childhood (up to the age of six), even though their symptoms may not make their appearance till much later. The childhood neurosis may become manifest for a short time or may even be overlooked. In every case the later neurotic illness links up with the prelude in childhood" (1940, p. 184).

These issues were further discussed during the symposium on "Problems of Infantile Neurosis (see Kris et al., 1954). Anna Freud reminded the participants "that analysts used to debate for years whether a mental disorder deserved the name neurosis before the pathogenic conflict was fully internalized. Another suggestion was not to use the term neurosis before the divisions between id and ego on the one hand, ego and superego on the other hand are fully established." She stated her preference for the latter, the structural approach, adding: "But since there is today a very wide divergence of opinion as to when the personality structure is set up, this will still leave many authors with the concept of neuroses occurring in the first year of life" (p. 43). The approach adopted in this monograph seems to me to go a long way to place such problems as those referred to by Anna Freud and Hartmann in the proper developmental perspective.

Spitz expressed the following opinion during the discussion in relation to Anna Freud's comments above: "I do not have the time to go into the question of neurosis in the first year of life, something which I do not believe exists" (p. 55).

Greenacre referred to two different uses of the term "infantile neurosis": "one, meaning the outbreak of overt neurotic symptoms in the period of infancy, i.e., approximately before the age of six; a second, meaning the inner structure of infantile development, with or without manifest symptoms, which forms, however, the basis of a *later neurosis*" (p. 18). She explained that it was to this second meaning of the term that her paper was addressed.

Freud's final view is that the phallic-oedipal phase in children occurs in the period from two to five years. My own experience at the Hampstead Clinic confirms Freud's view concerning the timing of the "infantile neurosis." Perhaps the majority of disturbances characteristic of the infantile neurosis can be observed between the third and fifth year of age, while in a few cases the fully developed infantile neurosis appears somewhat earlier or somewhat later.

Among the many developmental processes taking place in childhood, some are particularly significant turning points for the development of the personality. One of the most important is, of course, the developmental conflict taking place at the phallic-oedipal stage, a conflict of which the infantile neurosis is an expression. These disturbances, as Freud has shown, are the fate of all human beings, and healthy as well as psychopathological developments will result from their favorable or unfavorable solutions.

It is to be noted that the term and the concept of the "infantile neurosis" have both traditionally been used to cover a normal and typical developmental conflict as well as cases of mental pathology in which "infantile neurosis" has a much more serious connotation. The differences between these two forms are in part of a quantitative nature, depending on the one hand on the intensity of the phallic-oedipal conflicts in different individuals, and on the other on the differing strength and vicissitudes of the preoedipal elements and their individual contributions to the oedipal phase.

This poses problems concerning the definitions of normality and abnormality, health and illness, which are beyond the scope of this paper. However, I am using the term to cover both groups of "infantile neurosis."

In the preceding chapters I have described how the developmental interferences, and the developmental and neurotic conflicts taking place during the earlier phases, form the background and prepare the conditions out of which the infantile neurosis can develop. These earlier occurrences may have determined, for example, important fixation points and canalized drive and ego development into certain directions. All this will to a considerable degree determine not only the form of expression of the later infantile neurosis, but also its intensity, its future fate, and the ego's ability to cope with anxiety and conflict situations.

In Chapter 5 I have referred to the infantile neuroses as conflicts of a very complex nature. They appear only when the child has reached the phallic-oedipal level of development. This implies that multiple and very complicated maturational and developmental processes must have taken place on the side of the drives, in the child's ego, and in his capacity for object relationships. This high degree of organization of all aspects of the personality explains the great complexity of the disturbances taking place. The infantile neurosis is, in my view, an attempt to organize all the previous and perhaps manifold neurotic conflicts and developmental shortcomings, with all the conflicts typical of the phallic-oedipal phase, into a single organization, into a single unit of the highest economic significance. This compromise formation is possible at this point because of the relatively high degree of development reached in several areas, particularly in that of the ego's integrative and synthetic functions. For these reasons the "phallic-oedipal" phase is in fact an essential turning point in human development.

The complexity and levels of performance now possible compel synthesis, integration, and structuralization to degrees that were not possible before. This phase is thus an "organizer" of the highest significance in human development.[1]

I further believe that by this time most of the essential elements for the building up of the personality structure both in its normal and psychopathological aspects have already been contributed by the experiences and the maturational and developmental processes, although there are some notable exceptions, namely, the contributions of sexual maturation at puberty with its physical and psychological implications. Although latency, prepuberty, and adolescence do, of course, contribute new elements to the development of the personality, their main contribution may consist in reshaping, recombining, and rearranging elements or reinforcing specific tendencies which are mostly already present. I refer here especially of course to the establishment of psychic structure and the processes of structuralization. The influence of latency, prepuberty, and adolescence on the final structure of the personality will be discussed further in Chapters 7 and 8.

If one examines the symptoms and disturbances produced as the result of the infantile neurosis, he is immediately struck by some marked differences between them and the classical forms of adulthood neurosis. Only very rarely is it possible to see in childhood something similar to a typical adult neurosis or a very well-defined character structure.

What is observable in the large majority of cases are not finished products in terms of character or neurosis but rather less well-defined, much more diffuse neurotic and character organizations. There is a feeling of fluidity, of lack of definition, of processes potentially capable of developing in several directions, the final line not yet having been decided upon.

On the other hand, even within these more diffuse and fluid clinical pictures, it is possible to distinguish different types or forms of expressions of the infantile neuroses. The large majority of them are of a mixed nature, in fact, a combination of two or more of the types I shall now describe.

[1] To use a term introduced by Spitz in his book *A Genetic Field Theory of Ego Formation* (1959).

In some cases the disturbances observable, the symptoms produced, clearly belong to the phallic-oedipal level. On the whole and in spite of the intensity of the conflicts and the amount of castration anxiety present, the neurotic battle will be fought at the oedipal level, without any important regressive moves taking place in libidinal or ego elements from the phallic-oedipal position. It is not yet completely clear to us which factors are decisive in determining the level at which the neurotic struggle will take place or the neurosis organize itself—at least temporarily—at this stage. A significant factor in this connection is the presence or absence in any given case of important early fixations at the oral and anal phases. The more important the early fixations the stronger is the backward pull on the drives that have reached the higher levels of development. Furthermore, the larger the amount of drive energy arrested at the early points the less strong and resilient will be the phallic-oedipal organization. Regressive processes may start partly as the result of the intensity of the conflicts at the phallic-oedipal level, partly as the result of a weak phallic-oedipal organization caused by the reduced amount of drive reaching the oedipal level, and partly because of the pull backward to the fixation points.

In those cases in which the most important fixations are at the anal stage, the drive energy will mostly regress to the anal stage of organization and try to find its path toward discharge and gratification there. If the ego objects to this, conflict starts anew at this level.[2] The disturbances and symptoms produced will in several ways betray their close connection with the regressively reinforced anal component instincts and the defense activity against them.

If the economically more important fixation is at the oral level, the process of regression will reach back to this level

[2] If the ego raises no objection to this type of early pregenital gratification, a form of perversion has established itself (in the case of an adult) or favorable conditions for it in the case of a child.

and the form of the disturbance and the symptoms produced
will betray the attempts at oral gratification.[3]

I have observed that the persons who fight their neuroses
at the phallic-oedipal level respond better to treatment and in
general have a better prognosis than those who have taken
the path of regression. Similarly, I have elsewhere (1963) expressed the view that the prognostic outlook is better when
the clinical picture observed is the result of regression rather
than of arrested development.

In practice all sorts of combinations of these basic types are
possible. Fixations at various levels may exist and instead of
massive regression only more limited ones to the multiple
early fixation points may occur, while some of the drive remains engaged in the conflict at the phallic-oedipal level. In
this case the symptom formation is an expression of the
multiple situation of conflict at all the different levels. The
anxiety observable will manifest itself not only in the form
of typical castration anxiety of the phallic-oedipal stage but
in more primitive forms which correspond to the earlier developmental stages.

In attempting to evaluate an infantile neurosis and the
possible developments arising from it, another important
aspect must be taken into consideration, namely, the point of
its development at which we are observing it. Thus, at the
very beginning the main situation of conflict is centered at
the phallic-oedipal phase. A month later the same child's
clinical picture may be completely transformed, the infantile
neurosis having by now organized itself regressively around
the anal or the oral component instincts. This is presumably
due to the fact that in this case the ego was not able to attempt a solution of the conflict situation at the higher level,
either because of the excessive intensity of the original conflict or because of the backward pull of the fixations.

The precise study of the fixation points at the earlier levels

---

[3] For a more complete description of problems pertaining to the question of
fixation and regression, see Nagera (1964).

has prognostic significance for the fate of the neurosis itself and for the form of expression that it will or may finally acquire whenever the conflicts cannot be sustained at the higher levels.

Two other significant factors contribute to the changing, fluid, and diffuse character of the infantile neurosis. One is related to the fact that all developmental stages up to the oedipal phase have been covered in a comparatively short period of time, a circumstance which implies a certain amount of overlapping of phases (two to three years, for example). In some children this overlapping is particularly marked, and a relatively complete differentiation between the various phases seems to take longer than in other children. Thus, an unusually large degree of overlapping can be observed for a longer period of time. I believe that this less clear-cut differentiation and the amount of overlapping and contamination that they imply partly account for the confused, diffuse, and fluid quality of many infantile neuroses.

The second factor relates to the fact that although at the time when the infantile neurosis occurs most conflicts are internalized conflicts (among the different structures or aspects of the personality), the child's dependence on the external world is still so large that external events may easily upset and alter the still unstable inner equilibrium. Thus in the attempt to adapt to significant external events important economic shifts may have to take place, and in this way the whole inner defensive structure against the conflicts may be left weakened and in need of reorganization. The situation in this respect is, of course, very different in the cases of adult neurosis, because the adult is no longer so dependent on the outside world and has more efficient means of coping with it at his disposal.

My description of the infantile neurosis can in its essentials be applied to both boys and girls. Nevertheless, a few words about the phallic-oedipal development of the girl are necessary to highlight some important differences.

The girl's oedipus complex is not as straightforward as it is in the boy. She must make an additional step to reach her final oedipal position, although she can be said to reach the phallic-oedipal phase at the same time as the boy does. As in the case of the boy, her sexual position at this point is a masculine one (phallic). The object of her masculine strivings, like that of the boy, is the mother, with the father as a rival (Lampl-de Groot, 1927; Freud, 1931). This constellation is for the boy the "normal oedipal position," but for the girl this is only "the first stage" of her oedipal development. She is required to take other developmental steps. Thus, she has to change her leading erotogenic zone from the phallus (clitoris) to the vagina. Similarly, she is expected to exchange the phallic-oedipal object mother for the oedipal object father. When she has finally given up the mother as the object of her phallic oedipal strivings and replaced it by the oedipal object father, she has reached "the second stage" of her normal oedipal development. There are, of course, many possible variations of the schematic picture described above. Clearly then, the phallic-oedipal development of the girl is much more complex than that of the boy, and the correct assessment of her infantile neurosis and of the type of conflict underlying it is somewhat more difficult.

CHAPTER 7

DIFFERENCES AND SIMILARITIES
BETWEEN THE INFANTILE AND THE
ADULT NEUROSIS
WITH SOME COMMENTS ON PREDICTION

The processes and changes described in Chapter 6 on the "Infantile Neurosis" make many contributions to the varying shape of the disturbances of childhood. Many other factors contribute in varying proportions to this ever-changing picture.

The period of latency, for example, usually introduces a pause in sexual development, which in most cases brings about a marked diminution of the intensity of the child's drives. There is little doubt that these inner economic rearrangements that take place favor some extremely important developmental steps. Latency facilitates, for example, the child's move from the attachment to the oedipal objects to an attachment to his contemporaries. Many of the conflicts may and will now be partly expressed in relation to the contemporaries and displaced onto them. The degree to which these processes are completed varies greatly from one child to another and partly depends on how far latency is interfered with by massive conflict situations of an oedipal and pre-oedipal nature. In most cases, in spite of these interferences, at least some of the usual latency achievements can be ob-

63

served, although sometimes only to a limited degree and with evident signs of frequent interferences. Consistent clinical observation of these stages seems to me to demonstrate that the latency achievements are completely blocked only in very selected and extreme cases. In the large majority of cases changes do take place and these changes enforce a reshaping of inner forces, of inner economic balance, in one way or another.

Similarly, the latency pause favors developments in the ego which frequently result in a more capable and a stronger ego organization. The additional defense mechanisms that become available and begin to operate are different from the earlier and more primitive ones. Clearly, in most cases the new possibilities in this area facilitate a better coping and at the same time enable the ego to function in improved ways. For example, in most cases the amount of denial diminishes greatly at this stage. This represents an enormous advantage because we know how much the excessive use of denial limits the ego's ability to perceive reality properly and consequently to perform at its best.

Other no less relevant factors are peculiar to development itself, for example, the enormous variations in the rate of development of different children. Even more important is the fact that development must simultaneously proceed on the drive and ego sides along many different lines,[1] and that there is a constantly changing interaction and frequently a confrontation in the form of conflicts between them. Development along these many lines cannot be expected to proceed evenly, and this circumstance makes for the infinite variations in the clinical or developmental pictures observable at any given time in any given child. Furthermore, much of the unevenness among the different developmental lines may disappear at later stages when development of lagging areas catches up. Clearly, with the disappearance of the previous

---

[1] For the concept of developmental lines, see Anna Freud (1963, 1965).

imbalance between the developmental lines, further changes in the personality will occur and contribute to the ever-changing developmental picture of the child.

The following is an example of how the different maturational rates of different aspects of the personality contribute to these changing pictures. At Hampstead we frequently see children who, when they are going through the anal stage, react to the anal component instincts in a particular way, that is, by using special defenses which give rise to a specific conflict and produce symptoms of a certain nature. This reaction is frequently referred to as an obsessional development or even an obsessional neurosis (which at this stage it is not). It is an interesting question why some children react in this way while others do not. Furthermore, when one follows the vicissitudes of such obsessional developments setting in at this early age, they by no means imply that an obsessional neurosis will later develop out of them. On the other hand, there are many adult obsessional neurotics in whom it is not possible to demonstrate or recover an early reaction of this type to their anality. A point frequently made by Anna Freud in the past referred to Freud's statement concerning the fact that children with precocious ego development react very strongly against their anal component instincts, frequently bringing forward obsessional mechanisms.[2]

Some of the children who show these transitory obsessional manifestations appear to emerge relatively easily from this situation, perhaps because these phenomena are no more than the expression of the ego's objection to whatever anality is present. In such cases the next developmental stage will force anality into the background and the obsessional defense will no longer be necessary. If such a child safely negotiates the

[2] Freud mentioned that the imbalance between specific developmental processes going on at the same time in the child can be very relevant for the development of obsessional neurosis; he said, for example, "I suggest the possibility that a chronological outstripping of libidinal development by ego development should be included in the disposition to obsessional neurosis" (1913a, p. 325).

anal phase without the establishment of fixation points at that level, one can feel certain that he is not liable to develop an obsessional neurosis in spite of the early use of the obsessional defense. Anna Freud has frequently emphasized this very point, namely, that one cannot assume that an obsessional neurosis will subsequently develop merely because obsessional mechanisms become manifest at the anal phase.

Conversely, a child with constitutionally strong anal component instincts, but without the above-mentioned precocious ego development, will not react as much to his anality or display obsessional mechanisms during the anal phase. However, should there be an undue environmental interference with the child's anal impulses, one may assume that the anal phase will not be satisfactorily negotiated and that a fixation point will be established, although no obsessional defensive manifestations will be observable at the time. Difficulties will arise only one or more years later, at the phallic phase, when the ego development has caught up. At this point the ego will object to the ensuing regression to the anal phase, and now an obsessional neurosis could possibly develop if some other factors not always clearly discernible are concomitantly present (strong ambivalence, etc.). In other words, it might well be that the child's ego at this later stage reacts to the anal component instinct (when regression takes place) in a way similar to that of the child with the "precocious ego development" described above.

Since it is clear that not all regressions to the anal phase (resulting from later conflicts) will lead to obsessional neurosis, it may be of interest to attempt to understand, both from the ego and the drive sides, the reasons for the different outcomes.

The symptoms, the abnormal behavior, the disturbances observed in any given child at any given time are the outcome of conflict situations of a very different nature and etiology; but in spite of this different origin, their form of expression is, in many cases, identical. This is perhaps not sufficiently taken into account in our diagnostic and prognostic considerations. Some symptoms or disturbances may be the result of one or more developmental interferences at any given time. Others are the result of specific developmental conflicts, while still others are due to the existence of active and unresolved neurotic conflicts stemming from the present phase or remnants from previous ones. In some other children the symptoms and disturbances present may be partly due to the attempt to solve the conflicts typical of the infantile neurosis (phallic-oedipal conflicts). Although the structural changes produced by the developmental interferences may have a permanent character, the symptoms due to the developmental interferences may disappear as soon as the environmental conditions creating them change; or with the child's further progression and growth they may be neutralized, left behind, and lose their effectiveness. Similarly, the developmental conflicts and the disturbances and symptoms arising from them are likely to disappear with the next progressive steps taken by the child. These manifestations are consequently of a transitory nature in most cases. Even the symptoms derived from more permanent conflicts like the neurotic conflicts frequently tend to change their forms of expression in childhood, depending upon the current phase of drive development, the ego's heightened awareness of the drives and its ability to deal with them, and the increasing demands of a superego that is becoming more and more of a structure in its own right. Thus, for example, the oral gratification of thumb sucking can subsequently express itself in the form of greediness for sweets and even later in greed for food, massive smoking, or alcoholism.[3] Furthermore, the symptoms and abnormal behavior resulting from all these simultaneous but very different types of conflicts tend to change greatly as the result of, and in relation to, the more or less constant external (environmental) and internal (maturational, both physical and psychological) changes.

[3] For a fuller description of the changing forms of expression of many of the symptoms of childhood, see Nagera (1964).

In adolescence sexual development introduces a maturational factor that can completely change the inner economy
and alter the shape of the personality. Not infrequently some
earlier basic conflicts are swept away by the contribution
made by sexual maturation. In many cases bisexual and pas-
sive-active conflicts may take a turn for the better in puberty.
We do not know with any degree of certainty which factors
make this contribution so important in some cases, while in
others similar early conflicts remain essentially unchanged in
spite of the pubertal changes. Research into the factors and
conditions that regulate the extent of the contribution made
by sexual maturation at puberty may prove extremely fruitful. Furthermore, many other psychological processes crystal-
lize around this basic maturational move and contribute
further to the complicated picture of the personality during
adolescence.

A no less important element in the changing picture of
these preadult disturbances is dependent on the fact that during adolescence many of the old and earlier conflicts become
temporarily reactivated. Sometimes these reactivations are of
short duration, like flashes in a pan, coming and going many
times during the adolescent process. The picture of confusion
and lack of organization observable at this stage is addition-
ally enhanced by the fact that any one of any number of the
early complexes can be reactivated. They move into the foreground for variable periods of time (even for a few hours
only) giving way to any of many other early conflicts in quick
and disorderly succession.

Prediction under these conditions is a very difficult task,
but not always a completely impossible one. In many cases it
may be easier to establish some sort of negative prediction,
that is, to point to what is unlikely to take place because—
among other reasons—no specific vulnerabilities such as fixation points were established as the child passed through the
significant developmental phases. As Freud (1911b) put it: the

choice of neurosis "will depend on the particular phase of the development of the ego and of the libido in which the dispositional inhibition of development has occurred. Thus unexpected significance attaches to the chronological features of the two developments . . . and to possible variations in their synchronization" (pp. 224-225). For example, as said before, an essential precondition for the establishment of an obsessional neurosis is the existence of important fixations at the anal level, to which the drive development may regressively be forced back later if this type of neurosis is to develop.[4]

On the other hand, I also believe that predictions in the wider sense are feasible, that is, predictions covering a wide range of possibilities that are open to the personality depending upon the elements already integrated into it at the time of the phallic-oedipal phase. This is different from trying to predict where exactly development will settle, or what path of the many possibilities open will finally be taken. The latter prediction, though it may perhaps be possible in some cases, cannot, in my opinion, be made because of the many variables involved. There is no way, for example, to evaluate the scope of the contribution that sexual maturation in puberty will make, and how it will affect the final solution of earlier conflicts, rearranging the whole inner economy in unsuspected directions. Be this as it may, one gets a clear and strong impression that an essential aspect of development is to keep things fluid, to keep them on the move, allowing for as many contributions and recombinations of factors as may be of benefit to the personality for as long as possible. Anna Freud has long ago (1945) suggested that the seriousness of a disturbance in childhood should be assessed "not according to its damage to the activities or attitudes of the child in any special way or at any given moment, but according to the

---

[4] This is, of course, not the only condition required. On the contrary, certain others must be present and combine in specific ways to bring it about. Nevertheless, its absence (since it is a *sine qua non* condition) makes it unlikely, if not impossible, that such pathology will develop.

degree to which it prevents the child from developing further" (p. 136).

As the child grows older and as the phases are traversed on
his way to adolescence and adulthood, more and more becomes incorporated and fixed. In ideal circumstances all
these acquisitions seem to remain fluid, at least up to a point
(as if in the melting pot); but whenever the time is ready for
solidification, they will of course have to play a role. Obviously, all the available elements can be integrated in more or
less favorable combinations making the final outcome a more
or less desirable one. Here again, the study of the conditions
under which the final processes of structuralization take place
at the end of a long developmental chain may prove to be
another fruitful area of exploration.

One crucial factor in this respect is, I believe, connected
with the access to, and possibilities of, genital forms of discharge and gratification in relationship to an object, that is,
sexual intercourse. In trying to assess the results of analytic
treatment in adolescent cases I have made the following observations. Analysis is geared, among other things, to the
undoing of the regression of the sexual drive to early and
primitive forms of sexual organization. For many adolescents
true genital relationships are for a number of reasons not possible; and if they are possible, not without important interferences in terms of social organization, social disapproval
and guilt, quite apart from the fact that in terms of psychological maturity many adolescents are not at all ready for it in
spite of their completed physical sexual maturation.

In cases in which the genital, more mature and satisfactory
forms of sexual gratification are blocked, sexual satisfaction
is nevertheless sought and must come from somewhere. Such
adolescents may not always be able fully to abandon their
previous more primitive forms of sexual organization and
gratification, even when treatment has been successful. Further observations of some of these adolescents have shown
that when at a later stage gratification in "true genital terms"

is open to them, they can shift the whole of their inner economy in a most favorable way to adjust to these more mature and satisfactory forms of sexual gratification. At this point or shortly afterward they will abandon the regressed and more primitive forms (including masturbatory practices), as if automatically.[5] Thus these adolescents can easily convey an erroneous impression concerning the results achieved at the end of the treatment. Clearly, it is important to learn to assess the true state of their sexual economy, especially in terms of its potential to develop, its fluidity, and flexibility.

Some adolescents are obviously not able to make this move even if the possibility of object-directed genital gratification is available and conflict free, at least as far as the environment and society are concerned. We have not yet learned to identify with exactitude which adolescents have regained, through treatment, their potential to move forward and to make full use of the capacity to develop toward genitality at the appropriate time and which have not. The study of where such differences may lie and what they are based on will contribute to predictive studies in adolescence and help in the assessment of treatment results.

[5] In this connection "marriage" may to some extent reflect what I am describing. Clearly, it is a turning point for most people, either in a positive or a negative direction, but not infrequently it allows for great leaps forward in sexual adaptation.

CHAPTER 8

CHILDHOOD DISTURBANCES AS THE
BASIS OF ADULTHOOD DISTURBANCES

Freud explicitly referred throughout all his works to the adult neuroses as processes at the basis of which it was always possible to find an infantile disturbance.[1] This is still a basic hypothesis of psychoanalysis.

In *The Interpretation of Dreams* (1900) Freud said: "In my experience, which is already extensive, the chief part in the mental lives of all children who later become psychoneurotics is played by their parents. Being in love with the one parent and hating the other are among the essential constituents of the stock of psychical impulses which is formed at that time and which is of such importance in determining the symptoms of the later neurosis" (pp. 260-261).

In the "Analysis of a Phobia in a Five-year-old Boy" Freud (1909) referred to the fact that the neuroses of adults "could in every instance be traced back to the same infantile com-

1 It is of historical interest that in his early papers (1895, 1896), Freud excluded from this formula what he then called the "actual neurosis," that is, neurasthenia and anxiety neurosis as they were understood then. He believed that they did not necessarily have an infantile prehistory but were due to a combination of factors currently operating in the adult's life. At that time Freud referred to obsessional neurosis and hysteria as the "psychoneuroses." The first he thought to be the result of active experiences of seduction, and the latter of comparable passive experiences, which may have occurred early in life. It is well known that he soon abandoned this theory of seduction when he realized that fantasies of seduction in children are universal.

plexes that were revealed behind Hans's phobia" (p. 147).
Earlier in the same paper, he said: "When, however, an adult
neurotic patient comes to us for psycho-analytic treatment
(and let us assume that his illness has only become manifest
after he has reached maturity), we find regularly that his neurosis has as its point of departure an infantile anxiety such as
we have been discussing, and is in fact a continuation of it; so
that, as it were, a continuous and undisturbed thread of psychical activity, taking its start from the conflicts of his childhood, has been spun through his life" (p. 143).

In "The Claims of Psycho-Analysis to Scientific Interest"
Freud (1913b) wrote: "The normal sexuality of adults emerges
from infantile sexuality by a series of developments, combinations, divisions and suppressions, which are scarcely ever
achieved with ideal perfection and consequently leave behind
predispositions to a retrogression of the function in the form
of illness" (pp. 180-181).

In the *New Introductory Lectures* Freud (1933) referred to
"the fact that children [are expected] in a short space of time
. . . to appropriate the results of a cultural evolution which
stretches over thousands of years." In this context he further
said: "We are not surprised that children often carry out
this task very imperfectly. During these early times many of
them pass through states that may be put on a par with neuroses—and this is certainly so in the case of all those who
produce manifest illness later on. In some children the neurotic illness does not wait till maturity but breaks out already
in childhood and gives parents and doctors plenty of trouble"
(p. 147).

In *The Question of Lay Analysis* Freud (1926b) stated:
"The decisive repressions all take place in early childhood"
(p. 204).

In *Moses and Monotheism* Freud (1939) came back to this
problem: "A trauma in childhood may be followed immediately by a neurotic outbreak, an infantile neurosis. . . . This
neurosis may last a considerable time and cause marked dis-

turbances, but it may also run a latent course and be overlooked. As a rule defence retains the upper hand in it; in any
case alterations of the ego, comparable to scars, are left behind. It is only rarely that an infantile neurosis continues
without interruption into an adult one. Far more often it is
succeeded by a period of apparently undisturbed development. . . . Not until later does the change take place with
which the definitive neurosis becomes manifest as a belated
effect of the trauma" (p. 77).

Earlier (1916-1917) Freud had stated: "If a neurosis breaks
out in later life, analysis regularly reveals it as a direct continuation of the infantile illness which may have emerged as
no more than a veiled hint. As I have said, however, there are
cases in which these signs of neurosis in childhood proceed
uninterruptedly into a lifelong illness" (p. 364).

In some of his case reports, Freud presented clinical examples of the decisive influences of childhood on subsequent
neurotic breakdowns. In "From the History of an Infantile
Neurosis" Freud (1918) described the series of infantile disorders which lay down the predisposition for the neurotic
breakdown after puberty: ". . . every neurosis in an adult is
built upon a neurosis which has occurred in his childhood
but has not invariably been severe enough to . . . be recognized as such. . . . If our present patient had not suffered from
obsessional piety in addition to his disturbance of appetite
and his animal phobia, his story would not have been notice-
ably different from that of other children" (p. 99).

Freud frequently referred to the "developmental continuum" which human beings have to traverse before reaching
adulthood and maturity. He pointed to the important role
which failures in this development, especially in its early
part, play in later pathology. In his *Introductory Lectures*
(1916-1917) he wrote: "The studies on developmental me-
chanics by Roux and others have shown that the prick of a
needle into an embryonic germinal layer in the act of cell-
division results in a severe disturbance of development. The

same injury inflicted on a larval or fully grown animal would do no damage" (p. 361). Similarly: ". . . in view of the general tendency of biological processes to variation, it is bound to be the case that not every preparatory phase will be passed through with equal success and completely superseded: portions of the function will be permanently held back at these early stages, and the total picture of development will be qualified by some amount of developmental inhibition" (p. 339).

In "Formulations on the Two Principles of Mental Functioning" (1911b) he stated: ". . . the *choice of neurosis* . . . will depend on the particular phase of the development of the ego and of the libido in which the dispositional inhibition of development has occurred. Thus unexpected significance attaches to the chronological features of the two developments (which have not yet been studied), and to possible variations in their synchronization" (pp. 224-225). Further, he described (1926b) the ego as feeble and weak early in life, a situation which may be a determinant of illness in later life: "A feebleness of the ego of this sort is to be found in all of us in childhood; and that is why the experiences of the earliest years of childhood are of such great importance for later life" (p. 241).

In the Schreber case history Freud (1911a) said that "the forms which the neuroses assume retain the imprint of the course of development followed by the libido—and by the ego" (p. 79).

Jones (1955) quotes Freud as saying (in the Minutes of the Vienna Psychoanalytic Society of November 17, 1909):

"We expect it would turn out that the severe neuroses all have their prototypes in childhood life, so that we should find the kernels of the later neuroses in the disturbances of development in childhood. That is quite evident with, for example, the obsessional neurotics. This neurosis is almost mono-symptomatically concentrated on one point at the age of six to eight, and is already completely formed. It is a question whether everybody has not passed through a kind of elementary neurosis in childhood years, and whether the inter-relationship be not still closer than we imagine, so that not only the elements but the very prototype itself originates in childhood. The later neurosis may well be only a magnification of a product, which one can only call a neurosis, of the later or middle years of childhood. In that event we should have a clear view of the source of neuroses and should have to interpolate the 'elementary neurosis' as an intermediate stage between the nuclear complex [i.e., the oedipus complex] and the subsequent severe neurosis" [pp. 443-444].

CHAPTER 9

A DEVELOPMENTAL SCHEME: TOWARD NORMALITY, NEUROSIS OR OTHER FORMS OF DISTURBANCE

The diagram shown on page 78 is an attempt to approach the question of childhood disturbances, including childhood neuroses, from a developmental point of view. These earlier disturbances may finally result in any type of adult psychological disturbance or in so-called normality of adulthood.

The line of development which I have placed in the center of my presentation in this monograph is that leading to the adult neurosis[1] after traversing the infantile neurosis and all the earliest forms of conflicts which will influence and shape the latter's development.

The attempt to follow specially the line of development leading to neurosis is somewhat artificial, because the personality structure of essentially neurotic patients—or perhaps I should say, predominantly neurotic patients—usually includes other forms and types of disturbance as well. These are of course present in different combinations in any given patient.

Several years ago I treated a patient suffering basically from a severe obsessional neurosis; in the structure of this patient's

---

[1] The same can be attempted with any of the other lines of development leading to different forms of psychopathology either in the child or in the adult.

CHART I

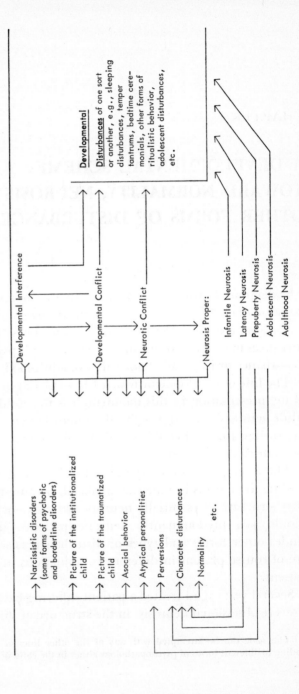

personality I could observe a combination of delinquent and perverse behavior, each existing in its own right. This patient demonstrated to an extreme degree what is by no means unusual in a large number of essentially neurotic or even normal people—that is, the existence of certain "pockets" of perverse or delinquent behavior.

The scheme outlined here provides for a similar approach to other possible outcomes of development in the human personality; it encompasses a range extending from normality to certain forms of psychotic disorders, the disturbances known as character disorders, asocial behavior, perversions, the clinical pictures of the institutionalized or traumatized child.

The emphasis is shifted away from the symptoms and the different forms of expression of the disturbance and is centered on the types of conflicts and their possible combinations which underlie the symptoms. In this way it becomes easier to judge the true nature and severity of the disturbances and symptoms which otherwise in a more superficial examination may look alike even though the disturbances may have a very different degree of severity and therefore a very different outlook.

The approach presented here gives due attention to the developmental processes and forces in all areas of the personality (drives, ego, superego, object relationships); it enables the clinician to assess pathology against the appropriate developmental background; and it takes into account the ideal picture of normality.[2]

Consideration is given to the reasons for the frequent changes in the symptomatic façade of the childhood disturbances and the fact that these disturbances are the result of different types of conflicts of a very different nature and severity, each type having a different potential to influence

[2] Hartmann expressed himself as follows: ". . . and we all agree that an understanding of neurotic development is not possible if it is not based on a very detailed analysis and on precise knowledge of what normal development is" (see Kris et al., 1954, p. 32).

later development. Attention is thus paid not only to the current disturbance but to its significance for further development.

My implicit assumption is that a combination of different developmental interferences, developmental conflicts, neurotic conflicts, in different proportions, leads to the development of the specific forms of neurosis in any individual; that is, in the early years of life, it leads to the different forms of "childhood disturbances," including the infantile neurosis, and in some cases to the later adult neurosis with contributions added from the latency and adolescent periods. There is of course no end to the possibilities of combinations of all the factors involved in such developments. It must be noted, however, that the term "neurosis" has not been used to describe the early disturbances in children. This term has been reserved for the "infantile neurosis," which I consider to be the first form of neurosis, and of course for all the later possible forms of neurosis.

In evaluating the different types of disturbances manifested by children, the somewhat defective or brain-damaged must be singled out for special attention. In view of the fact that their egos are different and atypical, they will react to the different developmental stresses in atypical ways. Their "infantile neurosis"—and I doubt that this term is really applicable—can be extremely atypical and distorted in comparison with that of "neurotic" or normal children.

The line of development leading to the picture of the institutionalized child also can be attributed to specific forms of early developmental interference: a lack of the indispensable minimum of human contact, no proper opportunity for stable relationships, or absence of the necessary minimum of stimulation. No doubt, the final picture will also receive contributions from other areas of conflicts (developmental and neurotic conflicts, etc.); nevertheless, in view of the timing, type, length, and intensity of the developmental interferences and the areas affected by their specific forms, the personality of such children is on the whole decisively shaped early in life and shows the specific characteristics of this type of disturbance.

Interferences of a different nature will leave their imprint on the child's identifications. These in turn affect the establishment of a healthy superego structure capable of dealing with the impulses and needs of the id and of compliance with the requirements for order and law of any given community. When there has been interference with identifications, the line of development may lead to certain forms of asocial behavior on the basis of a defective or inappropriate superego structure. As can be seen in the diagram, other forms of asocial behavior may be more directly the outcome or attempted solution of some specific types of neurotic conflicts or neurosis proper or of a combination of several such factors.

I make no claim for the completeness of this scheme. Obviously there is much of which we are not yet aware, and more that we do not know. I also do not claim to know what combinations of factors will lead to what results, except in a few cases where we already have enough understanding of several early genetic aspects of such disturbances. Despite these limitations I nevertheless believe that this type of approach, if carried on systematically, may in due time yield new insights and greatly increase our understanding.

As can be seen in the diagram (Chart 1), contributions to the clinical pictures (listed in the left column) can come from one or more of the types of interference and conflict (described in the middle column). The study of these contributions—where they come from, their intensity, whether they are taking place in the present or were active in the past and have already decisively and sometimes irreversibly shaped the personality structure—helps to assess the seriousness of the disturbance, and, perhaps even more important, gives relevant clues with regard to its prognostic evaluation. Clearly, it will be easier to deal with asocial behavior resulting from neurotic conflicts than with asocial behavior resulting from a defective superego structure, itself the result of undesirable developmental interferences.

In the diagram there are arrows that seem to indicate a progression from the developmental interferences to the neurosis proper, but this is only partially true. While in general there is such a progression, it must be kept in mind that developmental interferences can be active up to adulthood, or rather up to the point at which development in the sense here used has come to an end. Thus an adolescent suffering from a severe neurosis—perhaps a continuation of the infantile neurosis—can at the same time be suffering from a number of developmental interferences and from the typical developmental conflicts of the adolescent phase. Some of the developmental conflicts may transform themselves into permanent neurotic conflicts, which sooner or later will be incorporated, integrated, and synthesized with the previously existing neurosis and thus make a further contribution to it. These further contributions come from the phase-specific adolescent developmental conflicts which were not favorably solved, perhaps because of the added difficulties created in this hypothetical case by the existence of severe developmental interferences.

It may be clear from the above description that though the scheme is meant to cover the developmental vicissitudes from birth to adulthood, considerations similar to those applied to development as a whole are equally applicable to each developmental stage, as I have done in the case of adolescence described above.

Again, for example, when the child has reached the phallic-oedipal phase and suffers from the infantile neurosis, there is no doubt that looking back to the previous phases of his development we can frequently see at what points, and what types of developmental interferences, developmental conflicts, neurotic conflicts have played an important role in the disturbances he may have shown early. Similarly, we may be able to ascertain the contributions they may have made to determine not only the severity of the infantile neurosis but even its shape and form of expression. At the same time it is essential to assess the child's present phase (phallic-oedipal, in this case) and to note what developmental interferences may be present, and how they will favor or hinder the resolution of the developmental conflicts specific of the phase the child is going through. Faulty solutions may produce undesirable remnants in the form of neurotic conflicts which at some point are incorporated into the developing neurosis. All these will of course influence and partly determine what happens at the later phases. In this way we try to differentiate between the characteristics specific to a given phase and its genetic determinants. This approach was suggested by Hartmann (1950a), who remarked that "it may help us to differentiate more clearly the element of genetic continuity from the element of phase specificity" (p. 16). In right column of the diagram I try to show the possible origin of the so-called developmental disturbances, for example, sleeping disturbances, some forms of ritualistic behavior, castration anxiety, the disturbances of adolescence, as the end product of one conflict or as arising from a combination of several types of conflict at specific stages. Developmental disturbances can be observed as late as adolescence, stemming no doubt from the developmental conflicts of the phase.

Obviously, the right column of the diagram lists phenomena of a very different nature because they occur at very different ages. For this reason the background of drive and ego development against which they occur is very different. In temper tantrums, for example, there seem to be no conflicts of a psychological or neurotic nature; the problem is rather one of maturational imbalance between the strength of the drives, the resulting affects, and the ego, the latter being unable at this point to cope, repress, bind, or otherwise deal with the drives and affects. Certain forms of improper handling of the child by the parents may act as a developmental interference and tend to precipitate tantrums. As is well known, tantrums tend to disappear as soon as the ego means of control develop, and especially the capacity to communicate, to bind, and to discharge by means of verbalization. In a temper tantrum the child's ego is overwhelmed by emotions which it cannot handle. In view of this fact it may be correct to assume that temper tantrums are somewhat in the nature of traumatic experiences and the ego therefore tends to move away from them as soon as better means of coping are available. The bedtime rituals characteristic of the latency period, on the other hand, are based not in a maturational imbalance but in typical psychological conflicts about masturbation which are dealt with by means of typical obsessional mechanisms. Thus different developmental disturbances are based in phenomena of a very different nature. The use of the same term to cover such a variety of manifestations is, to say the least, misleading.

If one thinks, for example, of the line of development ending in the formation of an important character disturbance by the time of adulthood, we can see by following the arrows in the diagram that contributions to it are made in some cases all the way through life including late adolescence. This is true especially in those cases in which the final character disturbance becomes established at the end of adolescence; it is then possible to follow the contributions made at the different stages by some of the developmental interferences, developmental conflicts, neurotic conflicts, and by the neurosis proper, including contributions from the infantile, latency, prepuberty, and adolescent neurosis.

It is hoped that a classification of emotional disturbances, especially those of childhood, may be the rational outcome of what I have termed here "developmental psychoanalytic psychology."

BIBLIOGRAPHY

Deutsch, H. (1944), *The Psychology of Women*, Vol. 1. New York: Grune & Stratton.

Freud, A., Personal communication.

—— (1936), *The Ego and the Mechanisms of Defense*. New York: International Universities Press, 1946.

—— (1945), Indications for Child Analysis. *The Psychoanalytic Study of the Child,* 1:127-149.

—— (1954), Psychoanalysis and Education. *The Psychoanalytic Study of the Child,* 9:9-15.

—— (1962), Assessment of Childhood Disturbances. *The Psychoanalytic Study of the Child,* 17:149-158.

—— (1963), The Concept of Developmental Lines. *The Psychoanalytic Study of the Child,* 18:245-265.

—— (1965), *Normality and Pathology in Childhood: Assessments of Development.* New York: International Universities Press.

—— & Dann, S. (1951), An Experiment in Group Upbringing. *The Psychoanalytic Study of the Child,* 6:127-129.

Freud, S. (1895), On the Grounds for Detaching a Particular Syndrome from Neurasthenia under the Description 'Anxiety Neurosis.' *Standard Edition,* 3:87-115. London: Hogarth Press, 1962.

—— (1896), Heredity and the Aetiology of the Neuroses. *Standard Edition,* 3:141-156. London: Hogarth Press, 1962.

—— (1900), The Interpretation of Dreams. *Standard Edition,* 4 & 5. London: Hogarth Press, 1953.

—— (1905), Three Essays on the Theory of Sexuality. *Standard Edition,* 7:125-245. London: Hogarth Press, 1953.

—— (1909), Analysis of a Phobia in a Five-year-old Boy. *Standard Edition,* 10:3-149. London: Hogarth Press, 1955.

—— (1910 [1909]), Five Lectures on Psycho-Analysis. *Standard Edition,* 11:3-55. London: Hogarth Press, 1957.

—— (1911a), Psycho-Analytical Notes on an Autobiographical Account of a Case of Paranoia (Dementia Paranoides). *Standard Edition,* 12:3-82. London: Hogarth Press, 1958.

———— (1911b), Formulations on the Two Principles of Mental Functioning. *Standard Edition*, 12:213-226. London: Hogarth Press, 1958.

———— (1913a), The Disposition to Obsessional Neurosis. *Standard Edition*, 12:311-326. London: Hogarth Press, 1958.

———— (1913b), The Claims of Psycho-Analysis to Scientific Interest. *Standard Edition*, 13:165-190. London: Hogarth Press, 1955.

———— (1914), On Narcissism: An Introduction. *Standard Edition*, 14:67-102. London: Hogarth Press, 1957.

———— (1916-1917 [1915-1917]), Introductory Lectures on Psycho-Analysis. *Standard Edition*, 15 & 16. London: Hogarth Press, 1963.

———— (1918 [1914]), From the History of an Infantile Neurosis. *Standard Edition*, 17:3-122. London: Hogarth Press, 1955.

———— (1919), 'A Child Is Being Beaten': A Contribution to the Study of the Origin of Sexual Perversions. *Standard Edition*, 17:177-204. London: Hogarth Press, 1955.

———— (1923 [1922]), Two Encyclopaedia Articles. *Standard Edition*, 18:235-259. London: Hogarth Press, 1955.

———— (1926a [1925]), Inhibitions, Symptoms and Anxiety. *Standard Edition*, 20:77-174. London: Hogarth Press, 1959.

———— (1926b), The Question of Lay Analysis. *Standard Edition*, 20:179-258. London: Hogarth Press, 1959.

———— (1927), The Future of an Illusion. *Standard Edition*, 21:3-56. London: Hogarth Press, 1961.

———— (1931), Female Sexuality. *Standard Edition*, 21:223-243. London: Hogarth Press, 1961.

———— (1933 [1932]), New Introductory Lectures on Psycho-Analysis. *Standard Edition*, 17:3-182. London: Hogarth Press, 1964.

———— (1937), Analysis Terminable and Interminable. *Standard Edition*, 23:209-253. London: Hogarth Press, 1964.

———— (1939 [1934-1938], Moses and Monotheism: Three Essays. *Standard Edition*, 23:3-137. London: Hogarth Press, 1964.

———— (1940 [1938]), An Outline of Psycho-Analysis. *Standard Edition*, 23:141-207. London: Hogarth Press, 1964.

Hartmann, H. (1939), *Ego Psychology and the Problem of Adaptation*. New York: International Universities Press, 1958.

———— (1950a), Psychoanalysis and Developmental Psychology. *The Psychoanalytic Study of the Child*, 5:7-17.

———— (1950b), Comments on the Psychoanalytic Theory of the Ego. *The Psychoanalytic Study of the Child*, 5:74-96.

———— (1964), *Essays on Ego Psychology: Selected Problems in Psychoanalytic Theory*. New York: International Universities Press.

———— Kris, E., & Loewenstein, R. M. (1946), Comments on the Formation of Psychic Structure. *The Psychoanalytic Study of the Child*, 2:11-38.

Jones, E. (1955), *The Life and Work of Sigmund Freud*, Vol. 2. New York: Basic Books.

Kris, E. (1950), Notes on the Development and on Some Current Problems of Psychoanalytic Child Psychology. *The Psychoanalytic Study of the Child*, 5:24-46.

———— et al. (1954), Problems of Infantile Neurosis: A Discussion. *The Psychoanalytic Study of the Child*, 9:16-71.

Lampl-de Groot, J. (1927), The Evolution of the Oedipus Complex in Women. *Int. J. Psycho-Anal.*, 9:332-345, 1928.

Nagera, H. (1963), The Developmental Profile: Notes on Some Practical Considerations Regarding Its Use. *The Psychoanalytic Study of the Child,* 18:511-540.

———— (1964), On Arrest in Development, Fixation, and Regression. *The Psychoanalytic Study of the Child,* 19:222-239.

Provence, S. & Lipton, R. C. (1962), *Infants in Institutions.* New York: International Universities Press.

Segal, H. (1964), *Introduction to the Work of Melanie Klein.* New York: Basic Books.

Spitz, R. A. (1959), *A Genetic Field Theory of Ego Formation.* New York: International Universities Press.

———— & Wolf, K. M. (1946), Anaclitic Depression: An Inquiry into the Genesis of Psychiatric Conditions in Early Childhood. *The Psychoanalytic Study of the Child,* 2:313-342.

Symposium (1954a), Problems of Infantile Neurosis, *see* Kris et al. (1954).

———— (1954b), The Widening Scope of Indications for Psychoanalysis. *J. Amer. Psychoanal. Assn.,* 2:565-620.

INDEX

Actual neurosis, 72
Adaptation, 15, 18
Adolescence, 50, 58, 68-71, 78
    disturbances, 78, 80, 82-84
Adult
    and child, *see* Child
    "developmental interference" in,
        38-39
    impact of defense activity, 47
    neurosis of, *see* Neurosis, Psycho-
        pathology
Adulthood, 70-71, 74, 77-78
Aggression
    and fixation, 38
    oral, 51-52
Aim inhibition, 49
Alcoholism, 67
Ambivalence, 39, 66
Anal phase, 23, 42, 44, 52
    and ego development, 65-66
    fixation at, 59, 66, 69
Anal-sadistic phase, 19, 23
Anality, 65
Animal phobia, 74
Anxiety, 18, 49, 57, 73; *see also* Cas-
        tration anxiety, Fear, Separation
    anxiety

Bed wetting, 31, 33, 52
Behavior
    asocial, 78-79, 81-82
    delinquent, 79
    disorder, 45
    perverse, 79

Bene, A., 11
Bisexuality, 39, 68
Bolland, J., 11
Brain damage, 80
Burgner, M., 11

Castration anxiety, 19, 44, 59-60, 83
Central nervous system, 14, 41
Character
    disorders, 78-79, 84
    formation, 43, 46, 49, 58
    traits, 38-40, 46, 49, 67
    see also Personality
Child
    and adult, differences, 38-39
    clinging to mother, 31-34
    inappropriate demands on, 34-36,
        41-42
    institutionalized, 18, 22, 27, 29, 78-
        81
    needs of, 28-30, 41
    readiness, 41-42
    traumatized, 78-79
    vulnerability of, 46
Childhood disturbances
    and adult disturbances, 10-11; *see
        also* Neurosis
    basis of adulthood disturbances,
        72-76
    developmental scheme of, 77-84
    early, 13-14
    hierarchy of, 9-10
    severity of, 69-70
    see also Conflict, Infantile neurosis,
        Symptoms

89

Colonna, A., 11
Complemental series, 25
Component instincts, 23-24, 45-46, 48-53, 59-60, 65-66
Compromise formation, 36, 53, 57
Conflict
    around adaptation, 18
    in adolescence, 68-71
    between child's drives and environment, 39-40, 42, 48
    and development, 14-16
    external, 39-40, 43, 48
    interaction with "peaceful" development, 16-17
    internal, 39, 43
    internalized, 39, 43, 48-53, 61
    in latency, 63-67
    neurotic, see Neurotic conflict
    part of development, 17
    passive-active, 68
    phase-specific, and developmental interference, 36-38; see also Developmental conflict
    reactivation of, 68
    transitory, 49
    see also Oedipus complex
Constitution, 16, 25, 66

Dann, S., 18, 85
Dansky, E., 11
Death of parents, 19, 30
Defense, 17, 53, 61
    against anality, 65-66
    against component instincts, 59
    and developmental conflict, 47
    infantile neurosis as, 26-27
    and neurotic conflict, 49-51
    see also sub specific mechanisms
Denial, 64
Depression, 29
"Depressive position," 25-26
Deutsch, H., 18, 85
Development
    arrested, 60
    atypical, 22
    concept, 14-19, 41
    differentiation and integration, 15
    external and internal factors, 25
    inhibition of, 75
    interaction in, 14-19
    "norm," 10

    normal, 17, 24, 28-29, 56-58; see also Normality
    organizer of, 57-58
    see also Ego, Libido
Developmental conflicts, 37-38, 67
    anal, 41-42, 45-46
    concept, 41-47
    and infantile neurosis, 57
    and neurosis, 78-84
    and neurotic conflict, 48-49
    of oedipal-phallic phase, 56-57
    phallic, 43-44
Developmental continuum, 74-75
Developmental disturbances, 78-84
Developmental interference, 17, 28-40, 47
    definition, 28
    and developmental conflict, 41-42, 67
    and developmental phases, 19, 29, 36-37, 41
    gross (irreversible), 29, 37, 43
    and infantile neurosis, 57
    and neurosis, 78-84
Developmental lines, 77-84
    imbalance, 64-65
    toward neurosis, 77-84
Developmental Profile, 48
Developmental psychology, psychoanalytic, 13-19, 84
Diagnosis, 9, 66
Diarrhea, 31, 33
Displacement, 49
Dog phobia, 51-52

Edgcumbe, R., 11
Ego, 33-34, 39, 55, 79
    and affect, 83-84
    awareness and drive interest, 44
    conflict-free sphere, 15-18, 49
    development, 15-19, 65-66
    and developmental conflict, 42-43, 47
    and developmental interference, 36-37
    faulty development, 9
    hereditary core, 16
    and infantile neurosis, 57
    in latency, 64-67
    and neurosis, 75
    and neurotic conflict, 48-52

and physiological maturation, 15
precocious development, 65-66
primary and secondary autonomy,
16-17
strength, 50
and strength of drives, 83-84
synthetic function, 57
Environment, 24-25, 28-29, 41-42
interaction with, 14-19
overemphasis on, 44-45
Events, 28-34, 61; *see also* Environment
Experiencing, 18

Fantasy
oedipal, 19
of phallic woman, 27
of seduction, 72
withdrawal to, 49-50
Father, death of, 19
Fear, phase-specific, 45; *see also* Anxiety
Feces, smearing, 52
Feeding
difficulties, 31, 34-35
fixed schedules, 28, 30
Fixation, 19, 23-24, 37-38, 46, 57, 59-61, 66, 68-69
Frankl, L., 11
Freud, A., 9-10, 17-18, 21, 24-25, 29, 39, 48, 53, 55, 64-66, 69-70, 85
Freud, S., 16, 20-25, 27
bibliographic references to, 85-86
on choice of neurosis, 68-69
disposition to obsessional neurosis, 65
on ego development, 17
on infantile neurosis, 54-56
on neurosis, 72-76
on repression, 73
Freud, W. E., 11
Friedman, M., 11, 46
Frustration, 17-18

Greenacre, P., 21, 25, 56

Hartmann, H., 14-18, 20-21, 25, 55, 79, 83, 86
Holder, A., 46
Hospitalization, 19, 28-30
Hunger, 30
Hysteria, 72

Id, 16, 39, 43, 55, 81
Identification, 16, 34, 40, 50, 81
Illness, 28, 30
Individual differences, 41, 45, 49, 53, 64
Infantile neurosis, 9, 19, 67, 73-74
and adult neurosis, 63-76, 78-84
concept, 13, 20-27, 54-62
and developmental conflict, 47
and developmental interference, 37
developmental sequence, 23
and neurotic conflict, 50
timing, 56
Inhibition, 53
of oral aggression, 51-52
Instinctual drives, 15, 19, 79
and developmental conflict, 43-46
and developmental interference, 36-37
and infantile neurosis, 57-62
and neurotic conflict, 48-53
see also Aggression, Component instincts, Libido
Intelligence and anxiety, 18
Internalization, 40, 43
Introjection, 50-51

Jones, E., 75-76, 86
Jones, G., 11

Klein, M., 20, 25-27, 87
Kris, E., 13-15, 17, 20, 25, 55, 79, 86-87

Lampl-de Groot, J., 62, 86
Language, 15
Latency, 58, 63-67, 78, 80, 84
Learning, 16, 18
Libidinal phases
overlapping of, 61
see also sub specific phases; *and* Libido, development
Libido
development, 9, 19, 24
and fixation, 38
and neurosis, 75
Lipton, R. C., 18, 29, 87
Little Hans, 23, 54-55, 72-73
Loewenstein, R. M., 14-15, 17, 86

Marriage, 71
Masturbation, 19, 36, 43, 71, 84

Maturation, 41, 43-44, 50, 57-58, 65, 68
  concept, 14-16
  imbalance, 83-84
Memory, 49-50
Mittelmann, B., 25
Mother
  and child's development, 24-25, 42
  depression of, 29
  pregnancy of, 31, 33, 35
Mother-infant, biological tie, 29
Motility, restriction of, 42
Motor development, 15-16

Nagera, H., 9, 39, 48, 60, 67, 87
Narcissism, primary, 17-18
Narcissistic disorders, 78
Neurosis, 14
  adulthood, 47, 72-76, 78
  causes of, 24-25
  child vs. adult, 21, 58, 61, 63-71
  choice of, 23, 69, 75
  and developmental conflict, 47
  and developmental interference, 37
  elementary, 75-76
  infantile, see Infantile neurosis
  and infantile neurosis, 54-56, 78-84
  latent, 39, 74
  line of development, 77-84
  and neurotic conflict, 53, 78-84
  proper, 36, 48, 78, 81-82
Neurotic conflict, 36, 38, 47-53, 67
  and neurosis, 78-84
Newman, L. M., 11
Normality, 14, 56-57, 77-79
  variations, 21, 37-38
  see also Development

Object relations, 9, 15, 19, 42-44, 79
  and infantile neurosis, 57-62
Obsessional mechanisms, 52, 65-66, 84
Obsessional neurosis, 23, 65-66, 69, 72, 75, 77
Oedipal phase, 9, 19, 30, 34, 38, 41, 82-83
  developmental conflict of, 56
  and preoedipal phase, 56
Oedipus complex
  of boy, 61-62
  central role of, 27
  a developmental conflict, 44

  and earlier disturbance, 19
  of girl, 61-62
  and infantile neurosis, 23-27, 56-62
  nuclear complex of neurosis, 54-55, 76
  and superego, 50, 53
  see also Conflict, Fantasy
Oral phase, 23-27, 44
  fixation at, 59-60
Orality, 67

"Paranoid-schizoid" position, 26
Penis, 43-44
Perception, 50, 64
Personality
  atypical, 78-79
    contributions to, 22-27
  development, 22-27, 37, 49-50, 53, 57-62, 69
  and developmental interference, 37
  and infantile neurosis, 57-62
  and neurotic conflict, 49-50, 53
Perversion, 59, 78-79
Phallic phase, 19, 24-27, 30, 34, 38, 41, 82-83
  developmental interference in, 36-37
  and infantile neurosis, 56-62
  specific conflicts of, 43-44, 56
  timing of, 56
Phase specificity and genesis, 83
Phobia, 55, 73-74; see also Animal phobia, Dog phobia
Prediction of future development, 66, 68-69
Pregenital phase, 24, 56; see also sub specific phases
Prepuberty, 18, 84
Prevention, 13, 38
Proctor-Gregg, N., 11
Prognosis, 60-61, 66-67, 81
Provence, S., 18, 29, 87
Psychoanalysis
  a developmental psychology, 13-19, 84
  widening scope of, 22
Psychopathology, 56-58
  assessment, 79-84
  genesis of, 23-24, 77-84
Psychosis, 25, 78-79

Psychosomatic disturbances, 31-33
Puberty, 58, 68-69, 74, 78; *see also*
   Adolescence, Prepuberty
Punishment, 19, 36, 43
Putzel, R., 11

Reaction formation, 46, 49
Reconstruction, 23
Regression, 32-33, 36, 69
   and ego, 66
   and fixation, 59-61
Repression, decisive, 73
Ress, K., 11
Rituals, 78, 83
Roux, W., 74

Seduction, 72
Segal, H., 26-27, 87
Separation, 19
   anxiety, 32
   of mother and child, 28-34
Sexual intercourse, 70-71
Sexuality, 68-71, 73
   infantile, 54, 73
Sibling
   birth of, 35
   death of, 30
Skin irritation, 30, 33
Sleep disturbances, 33-35, 78, 83
Speech, 15
Spitz, R. A., 18, 29, 55, 58, 87
Stimulation
   deficient, 18, 22, 28, 80; *see also*
   Child, institutionalized
   excessive, 18, 28
Stross, J., 11
Structural approach, 55

Structuralization, 57-58, 70
   and developmental conflict, 46
   and developmental interference, 38, 40
   and phallic-oedipal drives, 53
   see also Personality
Sublimation, 46
Superego, 19, 39, 55, 67, 79
   defective, 81-82
   and neurotic conflict, 48, 50-53
   precursors, 43, 50-53
Surgery, 30
Symptoms
   and conflict, 14, 21, 79
   early, 36
   formation, 40, 45, 49
   identical, of different origin, 66-67
   and infantile neurosis, 58-61
   and neurotic conflict, 51-53
   transitory, 67

Temper tantrum, 78, 83-84
Thought processes, 49
Thumb sucking, 67
Toilet training, 28-30, 41-42
Tonsillectomy, 19, 30
Trauma and neurosis, 73-74
Treatment
   prognosis, 60-61
   results, 71

Verbalization, 84

Waelder, R., 25
Walking, 15-16
Washing compulsion, 52
Weitzner, L., 11
Wolf, K. M., 18, 87

ABOUT THE AUTHOR

HUMBERTO NAGERA was born in Havana, Cuba. He received a Bachelor of Science degree in 1945, a Master degree in Music in 1947, and qualified as a Medical Doctor in 1952. He then worked for several years as a psychiatric resident at the University Hospital of Havana.

Dr. Nagera became the Editor of the Psychiatric Section of the Cuban Medical Archives, and himself published many psychiatric and psychoanalytic papers in Spanish, as well as a book (also in Spanish), entitled *The Education and Emotional Development of the Child* (1958).

In 1958 Dr. Nagera moved to London, where he continued his training in child and adult analysis. He has been associated with the Hampstead Child-Therapy Clinic, where he is at present the Chairman of the Profile Research Group, of the Concept Research Group, and of the Clinical Concept Research Group. He has contributed regularly since 1963 to *The Psychoanalytic Study of the Child* where six of his most recent publications have appeared. Aspects of his work have been translated into French, German, and Portuguese.